501 E LOOK & FEEL GOOD TIPS

Published in 2009 by
New Holland Publishers (UK) Ltd
London • Cape Town • Sydney • Auckland
www.newhollandpublishers.com

Garfield House, 86–88 Edgware Road,
London W2 2EA, United Kingdom
80 McKenzie Street, Cape Town 8001, South Africa
66 Gibbes Street, Chatswood, NSW 2067, Australia
218 Lake Road, Northcote, Auckland, New Zealand

ISBN: 978 1 84773 363 4

Senior Editor: Emma Pattison
Editorial Direction: Rosemary Wilkinson
Production: Marion Storz
Design: Paul Wright
Artwork: Paul Wright

10 9 8 7 6 5 4 3 2 1

Reproduction by Pica Digital Pte Ltd, Singapore
Printed and bound by Craft Print International Ltd,
Singapore

Disclaimer
The author and publishers have made every effort to
ensure that all information given in this book is safe
and accurate, but they cannot accept liability for any
resulting injury or loss or damage to either property or
person, whether direct or consequential or however
arising. Anyone wishing to embark on a new diet or
fitness regime should consult a doctor before doing
so. All facts are correct at time of going to press.

501 EASY LOOK & FEEL GOOD TIPS

CATHERINE MORTIMER

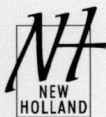
NEW HOLLAND

Introduction

It's all very well being a celebrity and having a nutritionist, personal trainer, make-up artist and stylist follow you about. But how does a real girl look good without this much help? I hope that by reading this book you'll be surprised how easy it is to look gorgeous and feel great too.

I've spent ten years interviewing celebrities and speaking to their stylists, hairdressers and make-up artists who work behind behind the scenes to keep celebrities looking great. I've learned no matter what your size, shape or colour there are enough sneaky beauty tricks out there to make the most of what Mother Nature gave you.

I've included everything I've learned, from make-up and fashion advice to ways to improve your well-being. I don't expect all 501 tips will apply to one person, but among the healthy recipes or step-by-step hairstyles, I hope you will find some that can improve your looks and your life.

I do my hair and make-up most of the time, I do an hour's exercise every day and I eat pretty healthily. But I have to confess that like a lot of women I enjoy a bar of chocolate and a couple of glasses of wine. On some days you'll even find me in a tracksuit with messy hair and no make-up. But I've realized that time out is important for your looks and life in general.

Which brings you to my story, I used to be your typical journalist, working late nights, gulping lunch at my desk and neglecting my health so I could meet deadlines. But then I started to develop back pain and in December, 2005, my car crashed in the snow. I was left with a slipped disc and no choice but to lie on my back for a year as part of my hospital treatment. It was a horrible experience but it made me more interested than ever in what it takes to look and feel good. It's where the ideas behind this book began.

I'm really passionate that beauty isn't just for people with big budgets or hours to sit in spas, flicking through magazines. Looking good is important to people who live in the real world, too.

I've chatted to hundreds of women throughout my career and they've shared some genius tried and tested tips with me. So inside you'll find a lively mix of celebrity style secrets as well as advice from people like you and me. Keep this in your bag and dip into it whenever you have a few moments. I hope my tips help you as much as they've helped me.

Enjoy!

Catherine Mortimer

FACE

1. SUN SEEKER

Swap sunshine for shade between 11am and 3pm, when the sun's at its hottest and you're most likely to burn. Sun damage is one of the biggest causes of premature skin ageing, so wear a sunblock with an SPF15 on your face (or higher during summer). You can save yourself buying two products by checking the label on moisturizers to see if they already contain sun protection.

2. TURN BACK THE CLOCK

Use a concealer in a shade lighter than your foundation to cover laughter lines and crow's feet around eyes. The lighter colour highlights areas that are wrinkled and gives the illusion of smoother skin. Finish off by blending foundation over your whole face and just like magic you'll look years younger.

3. SCRUB UP

Get a spa facial at home by whipping up a homemade anti-wrinkle polish. Mix 2 tbsp of almond oil with the same amount of porridge oats. Then using your fingertips massage it into your face every morning (avoid getting too close to your eyes). Rinse clean with warm water and pat dry with a towel.

4. MAKE-UP MASTERCLASS

Book an appointment with a make-up artist at a beauty counter for free make-up advice. He or she will be able to show you how to use products properly and recommend what suits you best. It's also worth going along to update your knowledge of new products and replace bits and bobs in your make-up bag that have seen better days.

5. LIP SERVICE

Oscar winner Halle Berry has a trick up her sleeve for getting the perfect pink pout when she hasn't got her professional make-up team to hand. The star applies red lippy then wipes it off and applies clear lip gloss. The subtle hint of colour is enough to pass off as a different lip colour.

6. BRIGHT EYES

Gently massaging either side of the bridge of your nose in the morning can get rid of fluid retention and reduce puffiness around eyes. Place two fingers on the top of each side of your nose, then using slow movements gently sweep fingers down and off the tip of your nose. Repeat ten times.

7. SMART SNACKING

Nibble on raw fruit and vegetables rather than crisps or sweets to boost valuable nutrients needed for the health of your hair, skin, nails and teeth. Cutting out junk food, which is highly processed and stripped of goodness, will boost your antioxidant intake and act like a gentle detox for your body. If you've got a juicer then have fun inventing smoothies to help keep you away from the biscuit tin.

8. SHINY SKIN

Instead of using powder to cover blemishes, switch to a light textured foundation. Powder settles in every tiny crease of your skin and highlights wrinkles dramatically. Choose a foundation that compliments your skin tone (see tip 16) and apply lightly to avoid overloading your skin.

9. SNOW WHITE

Did you know your choice of lipstick affects how white your teeth look? Pick your lip colour with care and your pearly whites will look amazing. Shades of pink achieve a white smile but avoid orange and brown tones, which make teeth look more yellow.

10. FACE-FIXER

Help a puffy face with a minute of massage. Place your hands either side of your head on the nape of the neck. Turn palms up towards the ceiling and thumbs down towards the front of the throat. (Your hands should be loosely 'locked' at the sides of your neck but thumbs shouldn't touch or you're gripping too tight.) Using gliding movements, work hands from the top of your neck to your collarbone. Repeat five times.

11. UNDER COVER

Celebrity make-up artists agree that a good light-reflecting concealer is an essential part of a professional make-up kit. Use it beneath eyes, on the sides of your nose, at the corners of your mouth, over fine expression lines and to help cover dark patches. It will hide flaws and bring out the radiance in your skin by catching and reflecting the light.

12. GRIN AND BARE IT

Here's what you need to do to achieve a perfect smile:

- Brush twice a day with a toothpaste containing fluoride to prevent plaque building up on teeth.
- Floss between teeth every day to remove plaque that your toothbrush can't reach.
- Change your toothbrush every three months.
- Brush teeth for two minutes minimum every morning and night.
- Limit sugary and acidic food and drink.
- Visit the dentist every six months for check-ups and your dental hygienist every three months.

13. CLOSE CALL

Almost all eye shapes are flattered by emphasizing the outer corners to create a wide-eyed effect. If you've got deep set eyes or they're close together then avoid applying too much make-up on the inner corners.

14. SAY NO TO SUNBEDS

Now for the serious tip! Protect your health and skin by limiting your exposure to the sun and sunbeds. Fair enough they make you look tanned, but it's actually a sign of tissue damage. Both produce ultra-violet radiation (UVR), which changes cells in your body and can lead to skin cancer. The sun's rays have the following effects:

- UVA – produces sunburn and suntans (but to a lesser extent than UVB).
- UVB – the biggest cause of sunburn and suntans.
- UVC – the most damaging to skin but UVC in sunlight is absorbed by the ozone layer. UVC from artificial sources can damage eyes.

15. DOUBLE TROUBLE

Tackle a double chin by strengthening lower face muscles. Sitting up straight in a chair, place your elbows on the table in front of you. Make your hands into fists and rest your chin on your hands. Press your chin firmly down against the resistance of your fists and then relax so your chin is resting on your fists. Repeat ten times. (You'll feel your front neck muscles contracting, which is normal).

16. FIRM FOUNDATIONS

Consider your skin's texture when picking a foundation. If you've got greasy skin look for products labelled 'oil free' but if your skin is dry go for foundations that are moisturizing. Combination skin is a bit more complicated. You'll need to first work out whether you're skin is more oily or more dry, then choose products as explained above.

17. FISHY FACT

Studies show fish fights wrinkles. Oily fish such as sardines, mackerel and herring contain omega 3, essential fatty acids which feeds skin cells and fights the effects of ageing. Salmon also contains DMAE (Dimethylaminoethanol) and firms skin. Pregnant women should avoid larger fish varieties, like tuna, which contains mercury that may be harmful to babies.

18. KISS AND MAKE-UP

Never emphasize eyes and lips at the same time when doing your make-up. Top make-up artists say it looks too overpowering. If you're going for a strong lip colour, cover blemishes or dark areas around eyes with a concealer and then dust a light eyeshadow over eyelids.

19. PERFECT PEGS

Here's how to make your teeth whiter:

- Dental trays – custom-made to the exact fit of a patient's teeth by a dentist. The wearer pours hydrogen peroxide gel into the tray and puts it in their mouth overnight.
- Laser whitening or 'power whitening' – your dentist applies a concentrated bleaching gel to teeth and uses heat from a special light to penetrate teeth and draw stains out.
- Home bleaching kits – a cheaper alternative to dental tray bleaching (above). Instead of a dentist fitting a tray to your mouth, a standard size tray is sold as part of a pack from pharmacies.
- Whitening toothpastes – don't affect the natural colour of your teeth but they help remove staining, which improves the overall appearance of your teeth.

20. FOLLOW YOUR NOSE

Cleanse your nose thoroughly of oily pores and blackheads by using a mild soap, cleanser or gentle exfoliating face scrub. Apply it to your face using small circular movements and cover the sides, stem, grooves and tip of the nose. For skin that's extra oily or congested, wrap a flannel around your index finger and go over your nose in the same way once more.

21. STAR TIP

Broccoli, cucumber, peas, asparagus, beans, Brussels sprouts, cabbage, spinach and watercress are all on actress Goldie Hawn's shopping list. The star juices green vegetables in a blender and drinks a glass every day to fight wrinkles. Green vegetables contain lutein, a powerful antioxidant that boosts eye and skin health.

22. FANCY A FACELIFT?

Protein is great for skin because it maintains your body's tissues and stops your skin feeling rough and wrinkly. Without it you'd have poor muscle tone, brittle nails and weak hair. Whipping up a chicken stir-fry cooked in sesame oil with added linseeds is a great skin booster.

23. EYE SPY

Take care not to drag the skin around your eyes down when applying or removing make-up or moisturizer. Heavy-handedness can cause wrinkles. But having said that, try not to fall into the trap of slathering your eyes with super-rich creams either. Thick moisturizers also pull delicate eye skin down. Instead choose an eye gel and lightly tap it around your eyes.

24. UNDER THE KNIFE

If you're choosing a cosmetic surgeon, make basic checks as follows:

- Contact professional medical associations to confirm your surgeon is fully registered.
- Ask your surgeon for proof of his or her qualifications.
- Ask how many procedures like yours they've carried out before.
- Enquire if you can see photos of their work.
- Ask for a detailed list of surgery pros and cons at your consultation (that way you can take it away and make a decision in your own time).
- Remember, if you're in any doubt don't do it!

25. WRINKLE REMEDY

Botox is the better known name for Botulinum toxin, which is injected into face muscles to paralyze them and leave skin looking smoother. Growing in popularity, the treatment is used to relax fine lines and the idea is that if muscles can't move then skin can't wrinkle. Effects can last three to six months until the toxin is destroyed by the body. There can be initial bruising and you should always choose an experienced doctor or therapist.

26. LASH FLASH

Apply mascara from the base of your lashes, sweeping outwards towards the tips. Don't pump wands in and out of the tube because mascara dries out quickly when you push air into the tube. A secret tip from celebrity make-up artists is to bend the end of the wand at a right angle if your hand isn't very steady. Always wait five seconds before blinking once you've applied mascara to avoid it smudging.

27. CHEEKY MONKEY

For perfect blusher, choose a tone that matches your face when it's flushed after exercise. Then pick the right formula – powder for oily or combination skin and cream for dry skin. To apply, look in the mirror and smile to highlight the apples of your cheeks and blend in lightly.

28. BERRY NICE

Raspberries, strawberries, cranberries, blueberries, blackberries, you name it – berries are full of 'good' chemicals called antioxidants. They neutralize the 'bad' chemicals, called free radicals, caused by pollution and sunlight which damage cells and leave skin looking older (see tip 103). Berries have super high concentrations of antioxidants compared to most other fruits.

29. REST UP

Look after your face by relaxing as much as you can if you have a stressful job, demanding kids or you're prone to worrying. Relaxing facial muscles helps prevent wrinkles and aches and pains. Help face muscles loosen up by lightly tapping your fingertips around your eyes, forehead, cheeks and mouth.

30. GLITTER BALL

As much as you might love a bit of sparkle, go easy with it if you haven't got the youngest of faces. Foundation or blusher containing glitter or shimmer can draw attention to older skin, especially on faces and make you look older.

31. PUCKER UP

To get a plumper pout, use a lip brush or lipliner to finely outline your lips just outside natural contours before you apply any colour. Avoid opaque lipsticks which generally make lips appear thinner and try tinted lip glosses instead.

32. MASCARA MAGIC

Before applying mascara, always curl your eyelashes – nothing opens up eyes better. You can buy eyelash curlers cheaply from most pharmacies and it only takes a minute to clamp them onto lashes. Mascara goes on easier after curling lashes and it'll stay put for longer.

33. SUN-KISSED SKIN

Your best bet for adding colour to skin is to go for a fake tan to avoid skin damage (see tip 14). Salons offer spray-on treatments which give the best effect but can be expensive. Before you splash your cash, you can buy plenty of good self tans to help you do it yourself at a fraction of the cost. DIY tanning can be better because you can build up colour gradually and avoid waking up looking orange the next day.

34. DRINK DAMAGE

As much as you might enjoy a chilled glass of chardonnay or a warming whisky, try to drink in moderation. Alcohol dehydrates the skin and speeds up the ageing process. It can also flare up skin conditions and increases bruising.

35. PERFECT POUT

For plump, soft lips brush a damp toothbrush back and forth over your lips for a minute (but don't go too hard!). It'll scrub away dry skin as well as boosting circulation. Then slap on a lip balm to seal in moisture and form a barrier against harsh weather conditions.

36. ALLERGY ALERT

When you apply a new product to your skin there's always a slight risk that you'll react badly. Try a patch test somewhere out of sight and leave it for 48 hours so you have time to see if it agrees with you. Products labelled 'hypoallergenic' suggest they won't cause an allergic reaction. But there's not a single product on the market that can guarantee somebody won't be allergic to it.

37. SLIP, SLAP, SLOP

If you're desperate to turn back the clock, invest in a good face cream that contains retinol (a form of vitamin A which maintains skin) and coenzyme Q10 (found naturally in skin and prevents damage to collagen).

38. LAYING THE FOUNDATIONS

The number one beauty rule when applying foundation or concealer is to always remember to moisturize skin first and give it a couple of minutes to soak in. If you don't, your make-up won't stay put very long and products could look crusty or flaky.

39. RISE AND SHINE

Some people buy blotting sheets to mop up shiny faces. A cheaper alternative is to carry a few sheets of toilet roll in your handbag. Simply separate the two layers and place one over the oily zone of your face. Lightly press it down and lift away.

40. EYE TEST

When shopping for eyeshadow, try out new colours on the inside of your wrist. That's where skin is most similar to skin on eyelids and you can see what it will look like most accurately.

41. CHEEKY CHAPPY

Make sure your blusher matches your skin tone or the end result will look totally unnatural and over the top. Pale skin suits light beige or soft pink shades. Pink skin looks good with pale beige or peach. Yellow skin tones are best with honey or coral and black skins go well with auburn.

42. NECKS BEST THING

Necks are a dead giveaway of your age and they're often left looking wrinkly and saggy without the right treatment. Every time you moisturize your face or apply sun protection, work a little into your neck using upward strokes to help keep skin as taut as possible.

43. SPOT ON

If you suffer from spotty or oily skin you need sun protection that's gel-based. Face creams made from oily formulations clog up skin and make spots worse. Always check you have sun protection of at least SPF15 or higher on hot days (see tip 1).

44. EYE TO EYE

Celebrities love coloured contact lenses. If you've always wanted a different eye colour then pop along to your optician. He or she will be able to advise you about cosmetic contact lenses and how to use them safely.

45. OFF TO A FRESH START

To give dry skin some deep moisturizing, mix together 1 tsp powdered milk with 1 tbsp ground almonds, then add 1 tbsp honey and 1 tsp aloe vera gel (which you can buy in pharmacies). After stirring well, smooth over a clean face, leave for 10 minutes and wash off.

46. CAMOUFLAGE

If you have trouble hiding marks on your face, there's a big variety of cover up make-up on the market that's thick enough to disguise everything from thread veins to scars. Special ranges include heavy-duty concealers in several shades to suit all skin types. The trick to hiding blemishes well is to build up cover gradually and blend thoroughly.

47. TURN THE OTHER CHEEK

Did you know your cheeks have very few oil glands compared to the rest of your face? Dryness caused by harsh winter winds or strong sunlight will show here first. Use a good moisturizer before going outside to keep peachy soft cheeks. If you've got greasy skin go for water-based creams rather than oil-based.

48. FACE FOOD

Make yourself a face mask using two skin superfoods – avocados and carrots. Combine 1 mashed avocado, 1 carrot (cooked and mashed), 1 beaten egg, 6 tbsp cream and 3 tbsp honey. Spread gently over your face and neck and leave for ten to fifteen minutes. Rinse with cool water and pat face dry with a towel.

49. HIGH BROW

As women age their eyebrows fade in colour and lose their shape. Don't fill them in too thickly and avoid using dark eye pencils if you want a natural look. Instead go for a mid-tone brown eye pencil and outline brows softly.

50. SLEEPING BEAUTY

Studies suggest skin repairs itself mainly between the hours of 1am and 3am, making it an excellent reason to slap on plenty of moisturizer before you go to bed. It's not called beauty sleep for nothing!

51. AGEING GRACEFULLY

Skin gets thinner and fine veins begin to show with age. If you've stuck to the same foundation for ages then it might not be doing its job as well as it used to. Carefully match foundation to your skin type (see tip 75) and apply more heavily over blemishes.

52. TIME TO TRASH

Experts say you should change your make-up regularly to make sure you limit the unhealthy bacteria you put on your face. Mascara should be binned after three months, liquid foundation, concealer, cleanser and moisturizer every six months and pressed powder, loose powder, eyeshadow, blusher, lip gloss and lipstick every year.

53. LASHINGS OF GLAMOUR

False eyelashes are quicker and easier to stick on than you think. The secret is to trim them to the length of your own eyelashes before application. Always trim from the outer, longer edges and apply the glue thinly so you can wiggle them into place. Then leave them to dry for a full minute before applying eyeliner to hide the join. The best liners to use are very soft pencils that smudge a bit.

54. BIG MOUTH

You can get plumper, sexier lips naturally without resorting to surgery or make-up techniques. Many make-up manufacturers make lip gloss containing ingredients like ginger and chilli pepper that tingle and stimulate lips so blood rushes to the area and plumps them up.

55. SPOT THE DIFFERENCE

Cover up spots using a concealer with a narrow nib to help blend coverage precisely over small areas. Check it also contains a drying out agent such as tea tree oil or witch hazel to get rid of spots faster.

56. COLOUR CRAZY

Experimenting with eye colour can make you look young again and it's a fun way to jazz up your make-up. If you're fair skinned go for cool pastels, but if you're medium or dark skinned then choose rich colours instead. Start by applying the colour along the top of your upper lash line. Flick out at the ends and blend upwards to cover your eyelids, without going up as far as your eyebrows.

57. TONE UP

Beauty products are often formulated for different skin tones to get the best results. Check you're using the right category for your complexion.
Here's how:

- Light skin products are designed for ivory or porcelain skin tones.
- Light/Medium skin cosmetics suit rose beige, light olive, or ash brown faces.
- Medium/Dark skin products go well with yellow beige, medium olive or brown complexions.
- Dark skin products are suited to dark olive, bronze or black shades.

58. LIGHT UP YOUR LIFE

If you're going to be outdoors most of the day, apply your make-up in as natural light as possible (close to a window helps). But if you're going for a candlelit dinner bare in mind that low light can make strong shades look harsh so go for a more subtle look.

59. NOSEY NEIGHBOUR

Make the most of your nose with these clever tricks:

- Disguise a long nose by using a light foundation on the lower half and blending it into a darker shade on nostrils.
- Slim down a wide nose at the bottom by applying a little dark foundation just above each nostril and blending it into your regular colour.
- To narrow a nose at the bridge, dot a little dark foundation at the top of the nose and at either side of the bridge and blend in to your normal shade.

60. LINE UP

When you're using eyeliner always draw the line all the way across the length of your eyelid for the most flattering effect. Lining only the outside half of eyelids makes eyes look smaller and closer together.

61. GLOW GIRL

Make use of bronzing powder to give your face an extra special glow. Remember to apply bronzer on areas where you naturally tan – on your nose, forehead, cheekbones and a little on your chin.

62. SOFT SKIN

Vitamin A is fantastic for conditioning skin. Many moisturizers now contain this vitamin (see tip 37), but you can get it naturally by eating liver, carrots, mangoes, sweet potatoes, apricots and milk. Pregnant women should avoid taking vitamin A which can damage babies.

63. EXERCISE FOR GOOD SKIN

Exercise improves your body's ability to transport oxygen throughout your body. Aerobic exercise is particularly good for improving blood flow and oxygen to skin, helping maintain a healthy glow and keeping it firm and toned.

64. BRIGHT EYES

If you have pale eyelashes or eyebrows and can't be bothered to apply mascara and brow pencil every day then try tinting. It lasts six weeks and colours can be matched to your natural colouring. Always get tinting done professionally and have a patch test first to check for allergies (see tip 36).

65. FRUITY FRIEND

When you're browsing the face cream counter look for alpha-hydroxy acids (AHAs) in the list of product ingredients. The most researched AHAs include lactic acid (from sour milk) and glycolic acid (from sugar cane). Benefits include increased skin firmness and scar reduction.

66. SPOT ON

Tea tree oil is a great antiseptic and antibacterial but it should only be applied to skin – never drink it. It's effective for drying spots out in a flash and treating cuts and grazes so they heal without infection.

67. KEEP IT ZIPPED

Sharing the contents of your make-up bag means spreading germs and infections. Cosmetics such as lipsticks, mascaras and make-up sponges are breeding grounds for all kinds of yucky bacteria and eye and mouth infections. Don't pass yours around and when trying tester products stick to the back of your hand.

68. PROTECT AND PERFECT

Tackle crow's feet by wearing a moisturizer everyday with an SPF15 or more to protect skin from the sun. When it's really sunny wear sunglasses too so you avoid squinting which causes wrinkles around eyes.

69. SUNBATHING BEAUTY

Statistically, women who use fake tan are twice as likely to get sunburnt skin because they wrongly assume a fake tan serves as a base tan to protect them from the sun's UV rays (see tip 14). Fake tans with sun protection only cover you for two hours after a tan is applied and not for as long as your tan lasts.

70. PEEL AWAY THE LAYERS

Chemical peels are used to rejuvenate skin and combat the signs of ageing, scarring and discolouration. Chemicals are applied to your face to superficially burn away the top layer, revealing fresher-looking skin. Choose between superficial peels which can be done once a fortnight, medium peels done once a year and deep peels which are once in a lifetime treatments. Results are good but there's some risk of scarring and it can be painful. Always choose a qualified surgeon or therapist.

71. MAKE-UP MAGIC
To hide imperfections make-up artists highlight other facial features. For example, if you have thin lips then play up your eyes to take the focus away. Take a look at your face and don't be afraid to say what you think is your best feature. Then always emphasize it when you're doing your make-up.

72. SLEEPING BEAUTY
When actors have been in heavy make-up all day they know the importance of taking it off properly. The secret to having great skin is removing all make-up before going to bed. If you leave it on overnight it can cause spot breakouts and uneven skin tone.

73. MAKE-UP ON THE MOVE
If you're short on space for make-up in your luggage, pack the bare essentials – mascara, tinted lip gloss, cream blush, and cream eyeshadow (which can be applied with fingers, not brushes). A matt mousse foundation is also handy because you can blend it with your fingers and it leaves a powder finish. Always stick to neutral and pale colours which don't need to be applied precisely.

74. TWIST AND POUT
You can buy a good variety of long-lasting lippy but to give any lipstick staying power you must blot your lips. Apply a coat of lip colour, slip a tissue between your lips and press down, then apply a second coat. Your lip colour will stay put even when eating, drinking or kissing.

75. FINGER PAINTING

Selecting the perfect colour foundation is one of the most important beauty rules when it comes to make-up. Choose a colour that's as close to your own skin as possible and apply dots along the jaw line to check for a colour match. Once you're happy with it, buy it and when you get home you can play around with blending and standing in different lights to see how much you need for good coverage.

76. CHIC CHEAT

If you're running late, feeling hungover or can't be bothered to put make-up on then a quick trick is to throw on a pair of sunglasses and swipe on some lipstick or lip gloss. If it works for celebrities, then why not everyone else? Keep an extra set of shades and lip colour in the glove compartment of your car. It only takes five seconds to fake looking great.

77. SEXY EYES

To achieve dark, dramatic eyes, use a black kohl pencil to outline top and bottom lashes and follow with a black liquid eyeliner on the top lashes only. Sweep a little grey eye shadow over your eyelids and blend for your desired look. Be careful not to use too much or you'll end up more ghoul than glam.

78. PUFFED OUT

If your eyes are puffy from a lack of sleep there are lots of soothing eye gels on the market or gel-based eye masks which you pop in the fridge before placing over the eyes, but a cold flannel or cloth does the job just as well.

79. DAZZLE LIKE A DIVA

Eyeliner that's infused with tiny glitter particles is an easy way to add a touch of razzle dazzle to your make-up. Glitter pencils also add sparkle around eyes without looking over the top. The thicker the line you draw, the more dramatic the end result.

80. GOBSMACKED

When applying foundation avoid getting an obvious line along your jaw where the foundation ends and your neck starts. A good tip is to open your mouth when blending foundation around the bottom of your face. It exposes the skin under your neck so you can blend it under your chin.

81. BUDGE THE SMUDGE

If you've ever put lipstick on and somebody has pointed out it's rubbed off on your teeth, chances are you're not the first person and you won't be the last! Avoid it happening by putting your finger in your mouth after applying lip colour then close your lips around it and pull it out. Bingo! Lippy stained teeth will be a thing of the past.

82. LATHER UP

Daily cleansing is important for removing dirt and sweat so moisturizer doesn't just sit on top of grime. Ordinary soap can be too harsh for some faces, stripping away natural oils and upsetting the skin's PH balance. Try foaming cleansers or creams instead. Work them into your face before bed, leave for a minute and wipe off.

83. HAIR-RAISING

Stars who prefer not to go under the knife have a trick up their sleeve to make their faces look taut. Tightly plait a section above each ear and fasten the plaits together at the back of your head. Viola! A facelift without the pain.

84. SEEING RED

Try to avoid situations such as smoky rooms or bright lights that will increase eye sensitivity and make you want to rub your eyes. Soothe blood shot eyes with an eye wash. Going without eye make-up is wise but if you can't bear the thought wear a mascara for sensitive eyes. See your GP if redness remains after a few days.

85. HOOD WINKED

To enhance eyes that are deep set or heavily hooded, use a light eyeshadow under the arch of the eyebrow to open up the area. Then apply a base of eyeshadow over the entire eyelid. Finish off with a little colour to highlight the side of your eyelid so that when you open your eyes the colour can be still be seen.

86. MORNING GLORY

Before going to bed put your moisturizer and foundation in the fridge. If you have a puffy face in the morning it will be cool enough to calm it down and it feels wonderfully refreshing (great if you find it hard to wake-up in the morning!).

87. LOOK OUT

Getting the right eyeshadow to enhance your eyes works wonders for the look of your whole face. If you've got brown eyes then try slate blue and navy colours, for blue eyes look for taupes and if you're the owner of green eyes go for mauves and lilacs.

88. GO GREEN

Buy a concealer with a green tint if you blush easily – it will cancel out rosy cheeks and red blotches or spots. Most pharmacies stock make-up ranges which include correction make-up with green tones to counteract redness (see tip 46).

89. BLINK AND YOU'LL MISS IT

Wearing eye colour is a great way to help eyes look younger (see tip 2) but make sure you use a good foundation over eyelids first. It acts as a primer before adding powder eyeshadows. If not, powder will stick to creases and make skin look a lot more wrinkled.

90. KEEPING UP APPEARANCES

Consider having permanent make-up applied at a salon if you dread the prospect of being caught barefaced. Popular treatments include eyeliner and lipliner, which is applied with a tiny needle that plants pigment just under the skin.

91. GETTING LIPPY

Stop lipstick from creeping all over your face by lining lips with a matching lip pencil after applying lipstick. It prevents colour bleeding around your mouth, which shows up instantly with strong colours like bright reds or dark plums.

92. MOISTURE MUST HAVE

Apply moisturizer to your face in upward sweeping motions to pull skin up, rather than dragging it down and making it sag. Spend two minutes every day massaging your face to boost circulation. If your skin is oily then only use moisturizer on dry areas like cheeks and avoid your forehead, nose and chin.

93. ROSY CHEEKS

Blushing is a natural response to anxious situations and the key to stop cheeks going crimson is to relax. Hypnotherapy helps reprogramme your subconscious and retrain your mind and body to react in different ways to situations that cause you to blush. Have a few sessions with a registered and qualified hypnotist to get you started, then try a self-hypnosis tape or book.

94. SWEET DREAMS

Studies show the skin's ability to repair itself peaks at night – that's why you should use a night cream once you turn 30. They're usually thicker and contain more nourishing ingredients than day creams so they stimulate cell renewal much more and reduce the appearance of wrinkles. If your skin is greasy, then look for a light formulation that won't clog pores.

95. TIRED EYES

Line lower eyelids with a creamy white eye pencil. It may sound odd but it gives the illusion of opening up your eyes and makes them look bigger. It's great for covering redness without having to wear lots of eye make-up. Apply it to the inside corner of both your upper and lower lids for best results.

96. RED WINE

A small glass of red wine every now and then could help you look younger. Resveratrol, a chemical found in red wine, influences enzymes in the body which control the ageing process (but that doesn't mean drink it by the bottle!).

97. GO BALMY

Never apply lipstick if lips are chapped as it may aggravate them and make them look flaky and crusty. Instead use a medicated lip balm or petroleum jelly twice a day to lock moisture in and protect lips.

98. BAREFACED CHIC

If you're not a big fan or colour, keep make-up simple. For an Audrey Hepburn look, focus on covering flaws by blending light-reflecting concealer and foundation over your face. Dust over a little powder and sweep blusher on cheekbones. Then using a sharp brown eye pencil, fill in eyebrows lightly.

99. GLITZ 'N' GLAMOUR

Metallic make-up is an up-to-date way to glam up an outfit. Blend metallic eyeshadow over your eyelids (you can take it up to the brows if you want a dramatic effect). Line your upper and lower lashes with a metallic eye pencil and apply black mascara. Keep the rest of your face simple, adding only blusher to the apples of your cheeks and gloss to the lips.

100. HOLLYWOOD SMILE

Many celebrities owe their dazzling white teeth to veneers, thin sheets of porcelain or plastic moulded over teeth to change their colour and shape. They're the perfect solution for teeth that are crooked, heavily discoloured, gappy or uneven. The downside is they're very expensive. But saving up for a few visits to the dentist to fit veneers will totally transform your teeth for ten to fifteen years.

101. BROW BUSINESS

Brush eyebrows into place before plucking. If it's your first time, use a white eye pencil to draw the shape you want and then make sure eyes are symmetrical. Your starting point is the inner corner of your eye. Pluck towards the arch and then find the best place to end by placing a pen or pencil vertically in front of your nose with the tip pointing up. Then move the tip diagonally until it crosses in front of the outer corner of your eye. This is the natural end to most eyebrows and is the most flattering point for your face.

102. SOFT TOUCH
If you've got sensitive skin and find facial exfoliators too harsh then invest in a muslin cloth and use it to cleanse your face every morning. It gently exfoliates without irritating delicate skin.

103. HIGH FIVE
You've heard it before but you are what you eat. Limit damage to skin from the environment by eating plenty of fruit and vegetables (or at least the recommended five a day!). They're packed with vitamins A, C and E, chemicals that neutralize the effects of pollution and sun damage. It's worth its weight in gold.

104. PICTURE PERFECT
If you want to hide a big nose, get photographs taken from an angle slightly above you. Alternatively, you can slightly lower your head when somebody is taking a photo directly in front of you. It minimizes your nose and makes eyes look bigger.

105. MASK IT
Give skin a boost by doing a face mask every now and then. Pharmacies and beauty stores sell a huge variety to suit every skin type and problem. Choose between clay, cream or peel-off masks. Study the labels carefully because the wrong face pack will leave skin spotty, oily or dry as sandpaper.

106. SUN SAFE
Keeping your face protected from the sun is the best way to keep skin looking young. But if you want to add a healthy glow then buy a tinted moisturizer. They're a great combination product and come in a variety of shades to suit all skin types.

107. NUDE SCENE

All the rage with celebrities, nude lips give you a natural and well-groomed look. Neutralize the pink colour in lips by applying a layer of foundation, than add gloss that's got a tan tint.

108. LUXURY LINER

If you have trouble drawing a steady line when using eye pencils or eyeliners, a good trick to steady hands is to place a mirror flat on a table and lean closely into it. Rest your elbow on the table and draw close to the eyelashes in an outward direction.

109. SANDPAPER SKIN

Dermabrasion has become a popular anti-ageing treatment. It involves skin being 'sanded' by a machine and although you're given a local anaesthetic there can be some discomfort afterwards and recovery takes two weeks. Micro-dermabrasion is a less painful alternative where a machine bombards skin with thousands of sterile crystals, then a pump removes the crystals along with dislodged skin. Both treatments should be carried out by a qualified surgeon or doctor.

110. BREATH OF FRESH AIR

Having a good tooth-brushing routine is vital for oral health (see tip 12). But don't forget your tongue if you get bad breath. You can buy specially designed tongue brushes but your toothbrush is every bit as good. Brush your tongue as part of your morning and night tooth-brushing routine.

111. LASH OUT

Erase dark circles under eyes with a good concealer. Then sweep a soft neutral eyeshadow over your eyelids and up to your eyebrows for the perfect canvas for black liquid eyeliner and mascara. It really makes eyes stand out and your make-up will still look natural.

BODY

112. CALORIE COUNT
To stay in shape you have to consume the same calories you burn off. To lose weight you need to take in less calories than you burn off. Daily calorie requirements can vary slightly with age but the average woman needs 1,900 – 2,000 calories and a man 2,500 calories.

113. STRIKE A POSE
Here's what to do to look your best in photos:
- Put one foot in front of the other, pointing your front foot at the camera and placing your weight on your back foot.
- Turn your upper body sideways to the camera.
- Hold arms slightly away from your body, resting hands on hips if preferred.
- Pull shoulders back and suck in your stomach.
- Finally, lift your head up and smile!

114. HANDY HINT
Swap hand cream for olive oil for extra soft hands and smooth nails. Apply a little before you go to bed and rub in well to dry areas. Slip on a pair of gloves to boost the effects of the oil (or socks work just as well). Leave hands to soak while you sleep. You'll wake up to silky soft hands.

115. TAKE YOUR TIME
Chewing slowly stops you gulping down mouthfuls of air with food so you don't end up feeling as bloated as a balloon. It also mixes saliva with food to aid digestion and give your brain enough time to register that you're full so you don't overeat.

116. SUN-KISSED SKIN

Before applying fake tan, it pays to exfoliate really well with a body brush, scrub or loofah mitt. It gets rid of dry and flaky skin so you don't end up with patchy colour. Work in fake tan cream or spray using small, circular motions and take your time. Most products come with protective hand gloves, or you can slather plenty of moisturizer on hands to act as a barrier cream. Wash hands thoroughly afterwards (orange hands are not a good look!).

117. GO GREEN

The aloe vera plant is a wonderful healer and soothes irritated or sunburnt skin. Look for it in after-sun lotions and moisturizers. Health stores stock supplements, which you can take daily to cleanse and calm an upset digestive system.

118. WEIGH TO GO

Toning up doesn't have to involve an expensive gym membership, you can do exercises with weights for free. Make your own hand weights by filling two empty plastic drinks bottles with water or sand. Carry them with you while you walk, swinging your arms for maximum effect. When you're used to them then increase the size of the bottle.

119. UNDER YOUR SKIN

Unfortunately, there's no easy way to erase broken veins. Intense Pulsed Light therapy (IPL) is where a spectrum of light is used to penetrate skin, leaving it looking smoother and firmer to help disguise fine veins. There's also Sclerotherapy, where veins are individually injected with a substance to make them shrink or disappear. Both require a course of treatments and may need top-ups.

120. SAVVY SNACKING

Create a nibble box by washing and chopping raw carrot, celery, button mushrooms and cucumber so they're ready to eat when you're feeling peckish. Like most salad vegetables they've got next to no calories so it's a great way of getting more vegetables in your diet without any fuss.

121. STANDING PUSH-UPS

Stand facing a wall with your feet a pace-width away. Place your palms flat against the wall at shoulder height. Slowly lean in towards the wall, bending your elbows downwards and breathe in. When you're upper body brushes the wall, push away and straighten your arms as you breathe out. Keep your back straight at all times. Repeat ten times.

122. BAKING HOT

Actress and model Elizabeth Hurley swears by home cooking for keeping her slim. A wise idea because preparing your own meals helps you keep track of what's going in your food. In restaurants you rarely know how many calories or what additives are in each course. So eating out is best as a treat because servings of food and drink are normally much bigger in restaurants than recommended portions (see tip 150).

123. MIND OVER MATTER

Change that way you think about exercise and see it as time for yourself each day, rather than another chore to cross off on your list of things to do. By focusing on exercise as time out from the pressures of daily life it can be a good mental and physical boost. Research shows that enjoying exercise helps you get results faster.

124. FUN IN THE SUN

A suntan is caused by an increased amount of protective pigment in your skin in an attempt to defend itself from the sun's harmful UV rays (which you probably know has been linked to skin cancer). Hollywood star Nicole Kidman maintains perfect skin by keeping out of the sun or covering herself in sunscreen and layers of clothing.

125. MILK IS A MUST

Experts say drinking milk helps burn fat. Rich in calcium, it plays a vital role in fat storage and breakdown. You can also top up your calcium levels by eating yogurt, soya beans, spinach, eggs, cheese and dried fruit.

126. HANDS UP

If you bite or pick at dry flakes of skin around nails, not only can skin bleed and sting but you can get nasty infections. Massage a little petroleum jelly or almond oil around nails after bathing or showering to keep skin soft and stop you being tempted to pick.

127. SLIM WITH SUSHI

Eat more Japanese food, it's generally low in fat and includes all the good foods you're always told to eat more of like vegetables and fish. Celebrity couple David and Victoria Beckham are big fans of the cuisine and order meals of sushi when they're staying in hotels.

128. BUST BOOSTER

Cheat your way to bigger boobs by brushing bronzing powder or body shimmer in between breasts to give the illusion of shadow and depth. Wear a push up bra to enhance your natural assets and choose tops that gather under the bust.

129. LUNGES FOR LEGS

Get in the habit of doing leg lunges if you want to perfect your pins. Stand with your feet hip-width apart, place your hands on your hips and pull your stomach in. Take a large step forward with your right foot, so it's underneath your right knee. Then return to the starting position and repeat on the other leg. Do five lunges for each leg and build up as you get stronger.

130. PAINT JOB

A base coat protects colour from staining nails and gives you a nice even surface for painting. Use three strokes on each nail for the best effect. Brush a stroke of colour along the centre of your nail first, painting towards the tip, then with your next stroke paint along the left side and then do the right side last. Let the first coat dry completely before applying a second. Don't worry if you make a mistake, just rub with a cotton bud dipped in nail varnish remover.

131. SNACK ATTACK

Celebrities are advised by their personal trainers to eat at least every three hours to stay slim. Supermodel Cindy Crawford and Hollywood actor Matthew McConaughey are among the stars who snack between meals. Going for long periods without munching on something slows down your metabolism because your body thinks it's starving and stores what you eat, rather than burning it off.

132. SIX PACK

Lie on the floor with your knees bent and feet on the ground. Suck your stomach muscles in towards your belly button. Slowly lift one leg and extend it so it's straight and hovering just above the floor. Bend your knee and bring the same leg towards your chest, hold for a few seconds and lower it to the start position without letting it touch the floor. Repeat 15 times on each leg.

133. BRUSH UP

Hundreds of beauty products claim to cure the dimply skin caused by cellulite, but if only it was true then we'd save so much time and hard work. The best way to tackle cellulite is to boost your circulation to help your body use up fat stores and flush out toxins. Buy a natural firm-bristled brush and take two minutes each day to brush skin before showering or bathing. Brush all over your body going in the direction of your heart using light strokes.

134. CAT POSE

Copying the way a cat stretches is great for aching backs. Kneel on all fours with knees hip-width apart and slowly drop your head and arch into a hump. Now reverse it and lift your head, let your lower back drop gently and stick you bum out. Slowly repeat three times but don't strain yourself. If pain persists book an appointment for a consultation with an osteopath or physiotherapist.

135. FAT'S LIFE

Replace saturated fat with monounsaturated fats (see tip 152) which lower bad cholesterol levels and increase good cholesterol. Foods rich in monounsaturated fats include:
- avocado
- almonds
- Brazil nuts
- sesame oil
- rapeseed oil
- olive oil

136. STRESS AND STRAIN

Stretch marks occur when you lose or gain a lot of weight quickly and fibres deep down in the skin separate under strain. The fine scars look like purple, red or silvery lines. When they first appear, over-the-counter moisturizing creams with vitamins A, E and alpha hydroxy acids (AHAs) can improve the appearance of stretch marks (see tip 65). There's no magic cure but in extreme cases laser surgery can help them to fade.

137. SMOKE SIGNALS

Smoking is the biggest and most avoidable cause of illnesses such as heart disease and lung cancer. It also affects your looks by dehydrating skin, depriving it of oxygen and producing free radicals (see tip 28) that accelerate the ageing process. If you smoke, write down how much you spend on cigarettes every day for a week. Then work out how much smoking costs you every year. Think what else you could do with the money.

138. GO NUTS

Snacking on nuts is good for boosting your looks. The fats, proteins and minerals they contain help the body's maintenance of hair, nails and skin. But don't go overboard because they're full of calories.

139. DRINK UP

If you're trying to lose weight then don't let yourself get thirsty. Thirst signals are sometimes misread as hunger pangs. Keep your fluid intake up throughout the day and you'll feel fuller and avoid reaching for snacks instead of drinks. Regular visits to the water cooler can also help you think more clearly and make better decisions.

140. DIVE IN

Swimming is a great exercise for all fitness levels, especially if you're getting back into exercise or you're a pensioner. Water supports body weight and because it's 1,000 times more dense than air it provides up to twelve times the resistance you'd get working out on land so it's a good workout for your heart and muscles. Swimming for 30 minutes three times a week will tone you up quicker than you think.

141. TALL STORY

Good posture gives you a better shape and it's instantly slimming. Standing with your feet hip-width apart, close your eyes and imagine a thread attached to the top of your head pulling your body up towards the sky. Slowly straighten your body up, first your head, then shoulders and hips. Then when you feel ready open your eyes.

142. PHONE A FRIEND

When the snack cupboard is calling, pick up the phone and not a chocolate bar or bag of crisps. Chatting helps get your mind off cravings by cunningly distracting you long enough for the urge to pass. Eat only if you're still hungry after 20 minutes (and try to make it healthy!).

143. HEART OF THE MATTER

During exercise your heart rate goes up as you burn fat. The harder you work, the faster it beats and the more calories you burn. Calculating your maximum heart rate (MHR) allows you to check the intensity of workouts. Find your MHR by subtracting your age from 220. Aim to work close to your MHR for best results, but never work at maximum intensity.

144. SOLE SURVIVOR

Everyone needs a bit of TLC from time to time and your feet are no different! Soak them in warm water for five minutes (or better still just have a bath). Remove hard skin with a pumice stone or scrub (body scrubs double-up as good foot scrubs). Rinse and dry your feet, especially between toes, and massage in plenty of moisturizer.

145. WATER WORKS
Ladies, you may already know that before a period hormonal changes can make your body hold on to excess water. But did you know salty food is the biggest culprit? It can add as much as 3 lbs (1½ kg) of extra fluid, so stick to the recommended 6 g (¼ oz) or less of salt per day. Season food with pepper, herbs and balsamic vinegar instead of table salt and drink two to three litres of water each day to flush out excess fluid.

146. LEAN LEGS
If you have chunky calves or wear killer heels most days then stretching your calf muscles will help slim legs down and keep them supple. Try going up and down on tip-toes ten times to stretch your calf muscles. Another way to elongate legs is to stand on a step, let your heels hang off the edge and drop towards the ground for 20 seconds.

147. THE 80/20 RULE
Fad diets are short-term fixes that don't work because you can't keep it up forever – so weight piles back on. But more importantly the world would be a boring place if you couldn't have a treat when you fancied it. Stick to a healthy, balanced diet 80 percent of the time and treat yourself the other 20 percent of the time. Weight gain and weight loss accumulate over time, so it's what you do in the long term that counts.

148. DRESS UP YOUR DIGITS
It's easy to cover up chipped nail polish if you take your own nail colour with you to have a manicure at a salon. After you get home you can still use it to touch up chips and keep nails in tip-top condition (really handy if you're going on holiday after having a manicure).

149. STRETCHING THE TRUTH

Take a few minutes in the morning to loosen up and stretch out. Doing it in the shower or while dressing saves time. Stretching keeps you toned and supple so you can move as flexibly as a teenager (even if you're birth certificate says different!). It also helps improve circulation to all parts of the body to ease niggling aches and pains.

150. SIZE MATTERS

Hollywood actress Renée Zellweger says she stays in shape by eating the recommended portion sizes of each food group. Here's what they look like:

- 150 g (5 oz) potato is the same size as a computer mouse.
- 75 g (2½ oz) of meat, poultry or fish is as big as a deck of cards.
- 100 g (3½ oz) serving of rice is half a teacup.
- 1 medium piece of fruit is the size of your fist.
- 25 g (1 oz) of cheese is a small matchbox in size.
- 1 tsp of butter or margarine is the same size as the tip of your thumb.

151. REAR VIEW

Bum, butt, bottom, backside or booty… whatever you call yours if you want to tone it up or trim it down try doing leg lifts. Kneeling on all fours, bend your right knee inwards as if trying to touch your forehead. Then lower it back down underneath you before lifting it up and out behind you (the sole of your foot should be facing upwards). Repeat five times on each side.

152. FAT CHANCE

Nobody's perfect and having the odd high calorie snack is normal but watch out for saturated fat, which increases levels of bad cholesterol and puts you at risk of developing heart disease. Plus it's high in calories, which leads to weight gain. Limit foods high in this fat, which includes:

- butter
- double cream
- red meat
- cheese
- pastry
- crisps

153. BRAVE NEW WORLD

Experts say you should exercise for at least 30 minutes five times a week. But when it's a mission to get motivated (like in winter), give yourself a goal. A sponsored run, joining a new dance class or taking up a team sport will give you a target to keep you interested.

154. STAR TIP

Celebrities are singing the praises of goji berries. Similar in appearance to cranberries, they're packed full of antioxidants to help protect skin from the effects of ageing. Chinese medicine practitioners believe the berries also improve your circulation and metabolism. They come dried in packs or as a juice from health food stores and big supermarkets.

155. DIVE IN

If you have painful joints it can make high-impact exercise like running totally unbearable, but don't give up! Take a dip down at your local pool instead. The water's buoyancy cushions the impact of exercise on your joints so you'll be much more comfortable. Plus you have to work harder against the increased resistance from the water, which tones you up faster. If you can't swim it's worth trying aqua aerobics which usually involves using floats.

156. UP THE ANTI

Avocados are a rich source of vitamin E, an antioxidant that's vital for good skin condition and wound healing. They also contain an amino acid called glutathione, which strengthens your defences against heart disease and cancer. Swap mayonnaise for avocado in your sandwiches (it's just as tasty) and your skin will thank you.

157. GET A GADGET

Tone up all over by walking in weighted training shoes, especially designed to work muscles harder and burn more calories. Some ranges claim they also help circulation and cellulite. Good sports shops can fit you with a pair and show you the correct walking technique.

158. IT TAKES TWO BABY

Studies show that dieting and exercise regimes are easier to stick to with the support of a friend. Find a buddy who will join you on a healthy eating plan or visits to the gym. You'll find it harder to break good intentions when there's someone else to let down.

159. SLIM LIKE A STAR

Actress Cameron Diaz keeps slender by stocking up on high protein foods, which keep you feeling full. The star says she keeps a supply of eggs and tofu (soy bean curd) in her fridge when she's at home. Both are versatile ingredients that you can add to lots of dishes to feel satisfied for longer.

160. GOLD STAR

For every week you manage to stick to a new fitness regime or healthy eating plan you deserve to give yourself a treat. Successful slimmers say they rewarded themselves with prizes like a new book, a manicure or a new pair of shoes to keep them going.

161. BOOGIE ON DOWN

Dancing for an hour burns the following calories:
- ballroom – 200 calories
- latin american – 300 calories
- line dancing – 300 calories
- ballet – 250 calories
- belly dancing – 250 calories
- pole dancing – 250 calories

162. CRASH DIETS

Dieters sometimes restrict their intake of vitamins and fats, vital for healthy skin and hair, when cutting back on calories. Studies show fad diets lead to poor skin condition and rapid changes in weight can damage the skin's elasticity, causing saggy skin. Stick to a balanced diet if you want to drop a few pounds and aim for a healthy weight loss of 1–2 lb (0.5–1 kg) maximum each week.

163. TUNE INTO TOMATOES

Boost your intake of lycopene, a member of the carotenoid family (a group of naturally occurring pigments which give red, yellow and orange vegetables their colour – see tip 233). This super antioxidant is found mostly in tomatoes and it neutralizes the damaging effects of pollution, and sunlight, as well as protecting against some cancers.

164. ARMY TACTICS

Tone flabby upper arms with tricep dips. Sit on a chair with your hands either side of your bottom and fingers pointing forwards. Raise your bottom up and slide it forward so it clears the seat, then straighten arms. Gently lower towards the ground, then straighten your arms and raise back up. Repeat ten times. It's not an easy exercise but it's very effective. Aim to get low enough that you're upper and lower arms are at 90 degrees.

165. SPILL THE BEANS

Stock up on soya beans which help build and maintain the skin's collagen to keep it looking plump and elastic. They also contain high levels of plant oestrogen and magnesium, both of which help minimize menopausal symptoms.

166. TELLY ADDICT

Developing bad habits soon takes its toll on your waistline. It'll probably not shock you to know that sitting and watching too much television is bad news if you're dieting. Studies show people who keep weight off don't watch the box much. In fact, successful slimmers watch less than ten hours a week.

167. GI JANE

Most dieticians agree that low Glycaemic Index (GI) diets, which ranks food according to how fast blood sugar levels rise when you eat them, can help weight loss and weight control. Eating low GI foods keep energy levels steady and creates a feeling of fullness to combat cravings. A detailed table of GI rankings is available on the internet, in health books or at some GP practices.

168. BRONZE MEDAL

Give legs definition and a healthy glow by sweeping bronzing powder down shins and around the curve of your calf muscles using a big make-up brush. Dusting colour over pasty pins makes them look healthier and creates the illusion of toned legs (but without the gym workouts!).

169. SUPER SELENIUM

Big news with skin experts, selenium helps protect against premature ageing by working in conjunction with skin smoothing vitamin E (see tip 156) to keep hair, skin and nails in good condition. Foods containing selenium include:

- tuna
- sunflower seeds
- Brazil nuts
- selenium-enriched breads

170. COMFORT EATING

Bingeing isn't always about hunger, some people are triggered to overeat by their emotions and it's a way of eating often linked to low-self esteem, stress and depression. Sugars in sweet treats release feel good chemicals in the brain, which temporarily act like a high. Eat small meals and snacks regularly to stay satisfied and fight cravings. Before you eat that slice of cake, ask yourself if you really are hungry.

171. PRETTY IN PINK

Give nails a glossy finish with pale pink vanish, it looks natural and suits most outfits. Dark colours are perfect for evenings out but remember that the darker the colour, the more quickly chips show up. Brush a clear top coat over dark colours to avoid a disaster.

172. BURN, BABY, BURN

If you want to lose weight then don't let more than two days go by without doing some sort of exercise. Don't worry it doesn't mean strict boot camp routines. Any activity that makes you work up a sweat will get the pounds dropping off. Brisk walking, swimming and stair climbing are great if you've skipped the gym.

173. WHAT'S IDEAL?

Find out whether you're under or overweight by working out your Body Mass Index (BMI). Divide your weight in kilos by your height in metres squared. (For example, if you weigh 65 kilos and you're 1.6 metres tall: 65 divided by (1.6 x 1.6) = BMI of 25.39.)

- 16 to 18 – underweight
- 18 to 20 – slightly underweight
- 18.5 to 24.9 – normal
- 25 to 29.9 – overweight
- 30 to 34.9 – obese
- 35 to 39.9 – very obese
- 40 plus – morbidly obese

174. BARBECUE BITES

If you cut back on alcohol at barbecues you'll be saving on calories without even noticing. Stay in shape by swapping red meat for chicken and fish and filling half your plate with green salad before you get near tempting alternatives. Now you can go to barbecues all summer long without worrying about your weight.

175. VITAL VITAMINS

You've probably been told this before but getting vitamin C (found in fruit and vegetables) has an array of beauty benefits. It's a powerful antioxidant, responsible for helping build healthy skin as well as fighting off infection. Stock up on food high in vitamin C, which includes:

- kiwis
- blackcurrants
- oranges
- peppers

176. BOOBY PRIZE

Slouching shrinks your bust by a whole cup size ladies! Stop slumping by pulling shoulders back and keeping your chin up when standing and sitting. Proper posture will make your chest look twice as pert.

177. WAIST NOT, WANT NOT

Your pelvic floor, the band of muscle at the bottom of your pelvis, is crucial for supporting your lower back and maintaining a good posture. Strengthen it by imagining you're trying to hold a penny between your bum cheeks when you're walking.

178. BIG BREAKFAST
Studies show that eating breakfast helps to boost weight loss. But before you reach for that chocolate croissant, it only works if you choose low GI foods that release energy slowly (see tip 167). Try oat-based cereals, egg on toast or a yogurt smoothie which are all low GI and will give you enough energy for the day ahead.

179. TENSE AND TONE
Isometrics is the term given to clenching muscles to tone them up. It's super effective on saggy bums, which get weak if you sit down a lot and don't exercise them (like doing a desk job which pays the bills but it's bad news for bums). Try squeezing your bum muscles really tightly for the count of five, release, then repeat. You can do it anywhere and nobody will know, give it a go as much as possible.

180. SCRUB-A-DUB-DUB
Red goose-pimply skin on upper arms and thighs is often a sign of bad circulation and the result of built up fat and toxins. Mix together 3 tsp of granulated sugar with your usual shower gel or bath oil and scrub skin thoroughly. Rinse away and feel the improvement instantly.

181. SNAP HAPPY
Stick your tongue to the roof of your mouth just before you have your photo taken. It tightens lower facial muscles and lifts a double chin, perfect if you're worried about a podgy face in close-up photos.

182. BATHTIME BLISS
It can be tempting to soak in a mega hot bath when you're aching from a long day, but drop a few degrees if you want to keep great skin. Excessive heat can damage skin cells and leave it with less firmness and tone. Keep your eye on the time too, after 20 minutes it's time to get out or skin will dry out.

183. SHAPE OF THINGS TO COME

Designed to change the shape of your body, liposuction involves a narrow tube being inserted under your skin through a small incision to suck out fat from beneath the skin. Areas targeted include tummy, bums, thighs, hips, chest, chin and knees. The procedure is carried out under general anaesthetic and recovery is pretty painful. Laser Lipo is a new alternative that's less invasive and uses a laser to melt fat which then naturally drains away. Always consult a qualified surgeon if you're considering cosmetic surgery.

184. BREATH OF FRESH AIR

How often do you think about your breathing? Many people don't breathe in deeply enough to get all the health and beauty benefits that oxygen offers. Breathing slowly and deeply increases oxygen flow to the skin and helps you relax. Go along to a yoga class where you'll learn breathing techniques you can use all the time.

185. LUMPS AND BUMPS

If you get ingrown hairs after plucking, shaving or waxing, you can help the problem by doing some exfoliation as part of your bathing or showering routine. Work a body scrub into your skin, then wash away to help keep pores unblocked.

186. ZEST FOR LIFE

Make yourself a lemon scrub, great for softening and whitening rough elbows, knees and heels. Cut a lemon in half and fill with sugar. Place each half over your elbows, knees or heels and rub firmly for up to a minute. (If you've got sensitive skin then give this a miss.)

187. BEAT BELLY RUMBLES

Carry a bottle of water and a healthy snack like a piece of fruit or a couple of wrapped up crackers in your bag. It'll stop you being tempted to buy sweets or crisps while you're out and about when hunger strikes.

188. GREAT LEGS ON THE GO

Tone thighs in the cinema, on the bus or sitting watching television. Press your lower back against the back of a seat and press thighs tightly together to the count of ten and then relax. Repeat ten times.

189. DITCH DIETS

Chances are you're heard it said before but research proves that diets don't work. Small changes to your lifestyle like eating more healthily and exercising regularly will help you lose excess pounds and keep them off for good.

190. SKIN DOCTOR

Everyone wants good skin and occasionally you need professional help, especially if you've got persistent itching, flaking or a rash. A session with a dermatologist will uncover any problems and it'll stop you bankrupting yourself buying endless products in an attempt to sort out your skin yourself.

191. NO NIBBLING

Try these tips to stop nail-biting:
- Always keep an emery board to hand for when you have the urge to nibble.
- Spend a few minutes each day caring for your nails (like polishing them) to give you a greater sense of pride in your hands.
- When you feel the urge to bite, do something else with your hands like squeezing a stress ball.
- If you're really struggling, invest in a bottle of anti-bite nail polish from all good pharmacies. It's formulated to taste so disgusting that you'll keep fingers away from your mouth.

192. WATER FEATURES

Do your skin a favour and limit shower time to five minutes. Showers rinse the skin's natural oils away and strip it of the moisture it needs to stay soft. Washing hands also zaps moisture from skin. Place hand lotion next to the sink for a nifty way to keep hands hydrated.

193. PROTECT AND PERFECT

Slap on plenty of sunscreen 15 – 30 minutes before going outside so it can soak in properly. When you're on holiday, remember to reapply it after getting out the sea or swimming pool. If you're in a country close to the equator where the sun is stronger, get a higher SPF sun cream (see tip 1).

194. HANDY TIP

Check the label on your nail varnish remover to see if it's acetone-free which is less drying for nails. Plus look out for formulations with added moisturizers to help replace the moisture stripped away when you take off nail colour.

195. HELPFUL HERB

After a big meal your waistband can feel like it's going to burst at any moment. Sipping mint tea and giving alcohol and caffeine refreshments a miss will help prevent bloating and indigestion. Try it for headaches and bad breath too.

196. NAIL IT

White flecks on nails are caused by heavy-handed manicures, nail damage or a lack of the minerals zinc and calcium. The recommended daily allowance (RDA) for an adult is 15 mg zinc and 800 mg of calcium.

Foods with zinc include:

- meat
- shellfish
- milk
- cheese
- nuts
- seeds

Foods with calcium include:

- milk
- cheese
- yogurt
- tofu
- sardines
- spinach
- dried fruit

197. THE BIG FREEZE

It's not easy to keep stocked up with fresh fruit and vegetables when you're busy with kids or work, is it? So keep plenty in the freezer on standby. Frozen fruit and veg is frozen quickly after harvesting so it keeps most of its nutrients. Always follow the preparation instructions on the packaging and never refreeze.

198. DO YOU SIP SODA?

Aside from stating the obvious problem – fizzy drinks fill you up with air. The sugar contained in them rots your teeth too. Did you know just one can of cola has about 7 tsp of sugar? Many fizzy drinks also contain caffeine which causes irritability, sleepless-ness, headaches and loss of calcium.

199. BELLY BLASTER

Getting a trim tummy doesn't always have to be hard work. Manuka honey from New Zealand is the latest natural cure for bloated bellies and digestion problems. It's been proven to soothe sore tummies and can be found in all good health stores and pharmacies.

200. RAINBOW RULE

Piling up your plate with different coloured fruit and vegetables helps to make sure you get a big enough variety of nutrients for good health. Add food in the four primary colours – red, green, yellow and blue/purple.

201. SAY CHEESE

Visualisation is a powerful motivation technique if you want to lose weight. Close your eyes and imagine yourself looking slimmer and hold that picture for a minute before opening your eyes again. Repeat it whenever you're tempted to buy a bottle of wine or bar of chocolate to help you focus on your goal. A tip for people with serious willpower issues is to stick the most unflattering photo of yourself to the fridge door to remind you not to raid it.

202. OUT AND ABOUT

Watching your weight can be a struggle in social situations like dinner parties or romantic dinners. Plan what you're going to eat in advance by checking restaurant menus for the lightest option and calling ahead of dinner parties to offer to bring a low calorie option for yourself.

203. TUMMY TROUBLE?

Try including live yogurt and other probiotics in your diet to boost levels of good bacteria in your digestive system to stop stomach upsets. Stock your cupboard with plenty of prebiotic food (which feeds the growth of good bacteria) which includes cereal, bread and yogurt.

204. SHOPPING SKILLS

Never shop on an empty stomach. Research shows you're more likely to treat yourself to high calorie food and ruin good intentions. Make a list and stick to it. It's the only way to make sure you only have healthy foods in the house (and if it naughty nibbles aren't to hand then you're less likely to eat them).

205. TUMMY TRIMMER

Tense your tummy – whether you're walking to the office or shopping for a pair of shoes. Sucking your stomach in regularly helps to maintain the natural corset of muscles around your middle and it can improve your belly in as little as a week.

206. TEA TIME

Drinking a cup of tea can keep your diet on track and help you look younger. Tea contains antioxidants to fight the affects of ageing and manganese, a mineral that reduces cravings by maintaining steady blood sugar levels.

207. ALL FINGERS AND THUMBS

Get in the habit of filing your nails in one direction to keep them strong and prevent splitting. Filing back and forth in a 'sawing' motion causes nail fibres to split and flake which leaves them prone to damage.

208. HEY SAUCY!

Stacked full of hidden calories, sauces can sabotage the best healthy eating plan. Swap mayonnaise, which is loaded with fat, for fat free fat Greek yogurt mixed with a little freshly ground black pepper for extra flavour.

209. STAR TIP
A fitness gadget that's favoured by celebrities such as Madonna and Elle Macpherson is the power plate, a vibrating exercise platform. Studies say it challenges muscles to tone them up faster than normal weight lifting and exercise. The only drawback is they're very expensive. But don't worry because heaps of gyms have caught on to the trend so you can have a go without breaking the bank.

210. SIP AND SLIM
Drinking spirits with low-calorie mixers is your best alcoholic option. For instance a single measure of gin or vodka with a slimline tonic is only 50 calories compared to a bottle of beer at 200 calories.

211. BINGO WINGS
Tone up arms at home by gripping a can of baked beans or bottle of water in each hand (see tip 118). Then standing up straight with your arms by your side, tighten tummy muscles and slowly lift both cans up and out to shoulder level, then return them slowly back to your sides. Repeat five times with 30-second breaks in between each set.

212. CLEAR OUT
Detoxing usually involves drastic changes to your diet and unwanted side effects such as headaches, upset stomach and low energy. It's better to follow a healthy lifestyle all the time and that way you won't have to put your body through extreme changes. If you smoke, drink a lot of alcohol or eat junk food regularly then consider cutting back permanently.

213. SPEEDY SLIMMING

Being realistic, it's hard to squeeze in exercise with all the other commitments people have on their time. If you want to lose weight quickly then focus on jogging for 20 – 30 minutes three days a week. It'll get you in shape fast because it's high-impact aerobic exercise which uses a lot of calories and burns fat very effectively. If you have joint problems, try swimming instead (see tip 140).

214. FRESH AND FRUITY

Eat more fresh fruit and less dried fruit. When fruit is dried, the sugar content becomes more concentrated, so it tastes lovely and sweet but it contains more calories. A big handful of dried fruit can have as many calories as a plate of fruit salad.

215. TIME TO TONE UP

A 30-minute workout burns the following calories:
- aerobics – 342 calories
- boxing – 225 calories
- cycling – 283 calories
- horse riding – 142 calories
- running – 365 calories
- skipping – 286 calories
- swimming – 248 calories
- walking – 120 calories
- weight training – 378 calories

216. CATCH SOME ZZZZS

Skipping shuteye plays havoc with your weight. Lack of sleep interferes with a chemical called Leptin, which controls body fat and tells you when you're full. Sleeping less than six hours a night will make you snack more (remember the longer you stay up, the more likely you are to eat too!).

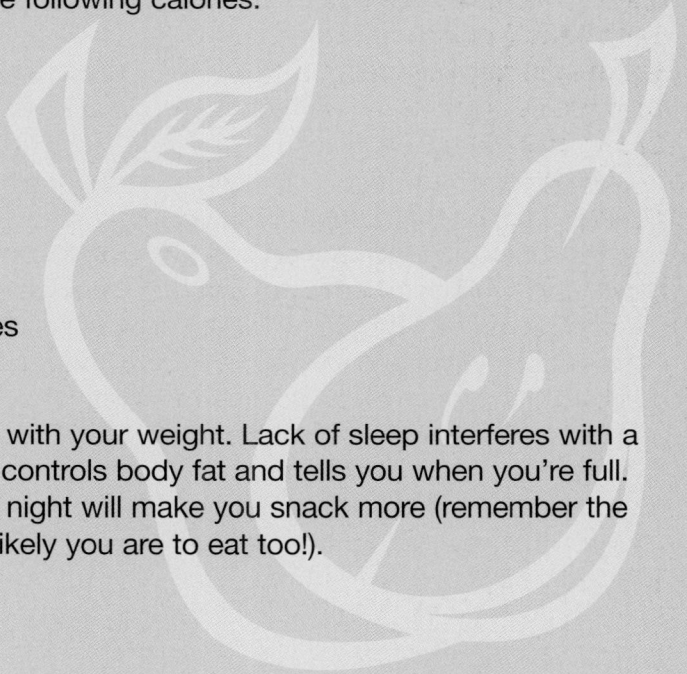

217. HULA HULA

Hula hoops were first introduced in America in the 1950s, but did you know they date back to ancient Egypt where they were first made from grasses? Although they're popular with children all over the world, adults are getting in on the action with hulaerobics classes and using hoops at home to tone waists and hips (and don't we know how stubborn it is to shift fat there!). Start off with two minute sessions and build up to ten minutes.

218. SENSITIVE SKIN

It can be a nightmare to look good if you've got skin that's easily irritated or you suffer from skin conditions such as dermatitis or eczema. Use plenty of emollient cream, which feels slightly waxy and works by providing a layer of oil on the surface of your skin to trap in moisture. Choose cosmetics and skincare products which are perfume-free and contain the least amount of chemicals possible.

219. VEG OUT

Vegetarians and vegans can be just as healthy as meat eaters. But to include a good balance of nutrients then make sure you get enough protein. The recommended daily amount is approx 45 g (1½ oz) for women and 55 g (2 oz) for men. Try chickpeas, beans or tofu (a tasty low fat substitute to meat made from soya beans).

220. THE F WORD

Keeping regular helps prevent big bellies and constipation and research says most people aren't getting enough fibre. Recommended daily intake is 20 – 24 g (¾ – 1 oz). Fibre is split into two types – soluble and insoluble fibre. But if you eat plenty of pulses and vegetables you'll get both groups of fibre.

221. PERFECT POSTURE
Back pain affects nearly half of all adults and it can change your posture so much that you look older. Strengthen core tummy muscles and strengthen your back with a quick tummy toner. Lying on your front, relax your legs and place your forehead gently on the floor and your arms out in front of you. Raise the opposite arm and leg straight off the floor and then lower. Then switch to the alternate arm and leg and repeat ten times with each pair.

222. WATER FALL
Check you're hydrated enough by looking at the colour of your urine after visiting the toilet. The more yellow or orange it is, then the more dehydrated you body. Drink at least two litres of water every day and aim for a very pale yellow colour.

223. DISHING UP
A really useful tip for checking you're eating a good balance of food groups is to divide your plate up at meal times. Fill half with vegetables, a quarter with carbohydrates and a quarter with protein. It's a great way of getting the right amount of different foods if you're not an expert on healthy eating.

224. FINGERTIP FASHION

If you bite your nails, false nails can be a good cover up. Here are the different types you can choose:

- Acrylics – tips are glued on (if extra length is desired) and then an acrylic mixture is brushed over nails, which sets hard over the top of tips. Acrylics are strong and long-lasting, but they're so thick they often look false unless attached by a professional.
- Gel nails – a special gel is first brushed onto the surface of the natural nail, then it's set under an ultraviolet light by a manicurist. Fingernails made from gel tend to look more natural than acrylic nails, but they're not as strong.
- Wraps – thin pieces of silk, fiberglass, paper or linen are cut to shape and glued or bonded to the surface of the fingernail. They're considered the most natural looking of all false nails but they're less durable due to the lightweight materials used.

225. VEG OUT

Losing weight shouldn't mean going hungry, just swap the sorts of food you eat so you consume less calories (see tip 112). High fibre food is a slimmer's best friend because it's low in calories and it bulks out meals, keeping you full for longer. Stock up on crudités, salads and fruit so you're ready when hunger strikes.

226. HEAVY WEIGHT TITLE

If you want to bulk up, don't be tempted to binge on junk food because it'll ruin your looks and health. Stick to a balanced diet and up your energy intake by 500 calories each day. Lifting light weights regularly will help you tone up the extra weight you gain.

227. GAME OF TWO HALVES

If you fancy a chocolate bar or a dessert has caught your eye on a restaurant menu then you don't have to say no. Life would be dull without treats, but the trick is to share them with somebody. That way you can half the damage to your waistline without missing out.

228. HEAD START

Splash out on a consultation with a personal trainer before starting a new exercise regime. It's money well spent because they're qualified to help you get to your goal as fast as possible without jeopardising your health or causing an injury. Most gyms offer a personal trainer service or can put you in touch with one.

229. SALAD SHOCKER

The last time you ate salad you probably thought you were being good didn't you? But some salads are higher in calories than a portion of chips or a slice of cake. Get salad savvy and pass on oily dressings and mayonnaise and limit nuts and cheese which are loaded with calories.

230. NICE NAILS

File nails quite short to keep them well maintained and healthy. Short nails go with all different colours and clothes. But the same can't be said of long nails, which can look overpowering when painted with rich colours or left tatty and yellow without varnish.

231. BELLY LIKE A BALLOON?

Check you don't have a food intolerance or allergy if you're bloated. Allergies tend to start straight after eating and can involve wheezing and rashes. While itchy skin or bloating are symptoms of food intolerance. If you suspect you're having these problems see your GP for tests.

232. ON THE BALL

Tone your tummy and strengthen core muscles with a Swiss ball. The giant inflatable ball is great for doing a variety of stomach exercises, which a gym instructor can show you. Begin by sitting on one for as long as you can to build up stomach strength.

233. FEEL THE CRUNCH
Carrots are a good source of beta-carotene, a naturally occurring pigment which gives colour to orange vegetables and has a strong antioxidant affect on skin. It can protect skin from sun damage as well as helping prevent some cancers. Eating carrots cooked with a little oil or fat encourages its absorption.

234. SOLE SURVIVOR
Hollywood star Demi Moore is a big fan of brisk walking. It works wonders for weight loss and toning legs and bums. The recommended daily steps for health is 6,000 and for weight loss it's 10,000 steps. Buy a pedometer, a small gadget you clip on your waistband, and aim for one of these figures.

235. GO ORGANIC
Research suggests organic fruit and vegetables contain more vitamins and minerals than produce sprayed with pesticides. Without chemical protection, organic fruit and veg produces more naturally occurring nutrients.

236. SLIM 'N' SAVE
Get a fitness DVD and workout from home as much as you like without paying expensive gym memberships. Cheap titles are normally available in charity shops or on Internet sites ebay and Amazon. If not then rent them from your local library.

237. GO BANANAS
If you suffer from water retention then grab yourself a banana, they contain potassium to help regulate body fluids and tackle bloating. If you don't like bananas, other potassium-rich foods include nuts, pulses, dried fruit and potatoes.

238. PACK IT IN

Save money and pack your lunch for work to stop you being tempted by the office sweetie jar or a piece of cake when it's a colleague's birthday. Filling up on healthy food is made much easier when it's at your fingertips, no matter how busy your day.

239. SWAP SHOP

Switch the brand of food you normally buy and get all your basics from your supermarket's healthy range. If you normally buy from the finest range it doesn't mean it's the healthiest choice (although it costs more!). By swapping to a healthier range you'll save heaps of calories without changing the types of food you eat.

240. PUTTING ON THE GLITZ

Ladies, when you're wearing a lovely dress and your hair and make-up is perfect, don't forget the rest of your body. Apply a little shimmer or tinted moisturizer to legs, arms and cleavage too help skin look glowing and blemish free.

241. KITCHEN CURE

Banish bloating by whizzing up a fruit cocktail to tackle water retention. Blend half a cantaloupe melon including its seeds with 1 cup strawberries with the tops removed. Cantaloupe melon is a diuretic that helps flush out excess water.

242. CRACKING UP

Wearing flip flops or sling backs exposes cracked heels. Exfoliate with a pumice stone or good foot scrub and apply lots of moisturizer before going to bed so it soaks in as you sleep. Put on some cotton soaks for extra softening before pulling back the sheets.

243. BOWLED OVER

Keeping a variety of fresh fruit handy makes you less likely to turn to junk food snacks when you're stressed, tired or feel like comfort eating. Invest in a fruit bowl and keep it well stocked to help weight control.

244. BACK TO BASICS

While you're in the shower remember to wash your hair before washing your back. That way you remove the residue from hair products that can stick to skin and cause spots. If you're already spotty, make sure you scrub your back to help pores unblock.

245. STREAKERS NOT ALLOWED

Recover from a fake tan disaster by scrubbing skin with a loofah mitt and body scrub (or salt if you don't have sensitive skin). It's the best way to remove streaks and blend away excess colour if you've gone a bit orange.

246. FLOWER FIX

Treat bruises with a little homeopathic help from the Arnica flower which studies show helps reduce swelling and heals damage to your body's tissues. Choose between tablets or creams from health stores and good pharmacies.

247. PERFECT PAINT

Painting nails when you're using the hand your write with (for example, your right hand if you're right handed) is one thing but when it comes to swapping to the other hand then things can get tricky. Avoid messy nails, sit at a table and rest your wrist on a surface to steady your strokes.

248. WEIGHTS ARE GREAT

Did you know that lifting weighs increases your metabolism permanently? Whereas aerobic exercise such as running only boosts it temporarily. Ladies can burn more calories without dieting with 2lb weighs (see tip 118). Lift and lower them to the count of ten to work muscles harder (ladies don't worry, you can't bulk up like men due to lower testosterone levels).

249. BRILLIANT BREAKFAST

Salmon Scramble. 260 calories. Place three cherry tomatoes under the grill for three minutes or until lightly cooked. Place two oatcakes on a plate with 120 g (4¼ oz) fresh salmon. Beat together one medium egg and 2 tbsps skimmed milk in a pan, gently stir and heat. When eggs are set, spoon over salmon and top with tomatoes.

250. WAYS TO WORKOUT

Here's how you can burn 100 calories:
- cycling for 15 minutes
- skipping for ten minutes
- having sex for 15 minutes
- scrubbing the floor for 15 minutes
- playing a physical game with your children for 20 minutes
- swimming for 20 minutes
- vacuuming for 30 minutes
- ice-skating for 20 minutes
- shopping for an hour
- do a fitness DVD for ten minutes
- washing the car for 30 minutes

251. DIVINE DINNER

Chickpea burgers. 273 calories. Finely mince together 120 g (4¼ oz) roasted chicken pieces, 50 g (1¾ oz) canned chickpeas (drained), half a small chopped onion and half a finely chopped garlic clove. Remove to a bowl and add half a tsp of finally chopped fresh sage and 50 g (1¾ oz) breadcrumbs. Beat an egg and use half of it to bind the mince. Spread 20 g (¾ oz) breadcrumbs over a large baking sheet and take a handful of mixture at a time, mould into burger shapes and coat in breadcrumbs. Grill for 7 – 10 minutes under a medium heat, until golden and serve with a green salad.

252. WOBBLY WAISTLINE?

Grab a friend and join a Pilates class which is popular with celebrities for keeping their tummies under control. The best stomach-toning techniques come from this form of exercise and it's easy to get results fast.

253. LEAN CUISINE

It's not always what you eat but how you cook it. Ditch frying for grilling, which requires less or no oil, and swap boiling for steaming to keep nutrients in tact (a metal colander over a pan will do the job if you don't have a steamer).

254. TAN FAN

Most fake tans contain dihydroxyacetone (DHA), which reacts with the skin's amino acids to produce a darkened colour within three to four hours. But if you've tried it you'll know you can end up smelling a bit like a biscuit. Thankfully, herb-based tans are now on sale from good pharmacies and beauty stores.

255. SWAP, DON'T STARVE

The key to losing weight is making sustainable changes but face facts there are some foods you just love! So if you can't live without tortilla chips, trying to cut them out entirely won't work. Find little swaps that work for you like changing to a reduced fat tortilla chip.

256. HIGHLIGHT HANDS

Nail varnish, like accessories, should compliment your clothes and match your make-up. Here's how:

- Clear, pink, cream or beige varnishes add a glossy well-groomed touch. Whatever your style, these natural shades always work.
- Red nail polish is ultra sexy and goes perfectly with red lipstick.
- Dark colours like brown, plum and purple complement dark eye make-up.

257. SUPER SPINACH

Add spinach to salads and sandwiches to pick you up when you're tired. Rich in folate, a B vitamin that plays a key part in the body's production of energy. These green leaves give you a boost and help your metabolism.

258. BEST CHEST

If your breasts have started heading south, there's not much you can do about it unless they're so bad you can look into surgery (which is painful and costly). But firming up the underlying pectoral muscles can help. Washing windows is a chore that's great for toning upper arms, upper back and boobs – and the bigger the movements the better.

259. ON THE MENU
Don't be afraid to ask a waiter or waitress for options that aren't on the menu when eating out. Request a salad instead of chips on the side of your meal, choose wholegrain rather than white bread and ask for salad dressing to be served separately. Having a glass of water with every course will also help you fill up by the time the dessert menu gets waved under your nose.

260. STEP BY STEP
If you struggle to motivate yourself to exercise (which comes to most of us at times!), take a tip from Hollywood actress Sharon Stone. The star sets herself small goals that are easily achievable, like walking up the stairs and parking a few roads away from where she wants to go.

261. EAT TO ENERGIZE
Oats contain more protein than any other cereal and they're a great source of B vitamins which help energy production and pick you up when you're tired. Choose porridge or oatcakes to give you a boost at breakfast time.

262. FRENCH FASHION
Great for keeping natural-looking nails, French manicures add a touch of glamour. Apply a clear base coat and let it dry. Then paint on two coats of pale pink nail polish and allow to dry. Using French manicure stencils (which are available from good pharmacies) hold close to the nail and apply white polish to nail tips. Then let polish dry before removing the stencils.

263. SPARE TYRE
Tone your tummy muscles by lying on the floor with your knees bent and feet flat on the ground and hip-width apart. Raise yourself up on to your elbows and pull in your stomach. Lift your right leg just off the floor and make little circles in the air with your foot. Swap feet and repeat ten times on each side.

264. LIGHTEN UP
Tackle yellow nails the natural way. Soak a cotton bud in natural lemon juice and rub a generous amount on to each nail. Leave to soak for a few minutes before washing hands and moisturizing well. Don't do this if you have sensitive hands or skin conditions.

265. CHOP! CHOP!
Make exercise more interesting by mixing up what you do each day. Superstar Madonna reckons she switches between pilates, horse riding and yoga. It helps the singer work different muscles to keep her in perfect shape without getting bored.

266. SUNSET SOLUTION
If you're sunburnt or you've been in the sun all day and your skin is dry and rough, then wash skin in warm or cool water (whichever is most comfortable) to remove any dirt or sand. Then apply an after-sun lotion to soothe the skin, cool it down and replace moisture. It helps prevent peeling too so your tan lasts longer.

267. FIGURE IT OUT
It's easy to cut 100 calories without dieting.
- Swap a croissant for two poached eggs on toast.
- Go for a baked potato with beans and salad instead of butter and cheese.
- Choose tomato based soups rather than cream.
- Swap a chocolate bar for an oatcake spread thinly with chocolate spread.
- Opt for a piece of fruit rather than a fruit smoothie.
- Fill half your glass of wine with fizzy water.
- Swap a large coffee made from whole milk for skimmed milk.
- Switch two chocolate biscuits for two chocolate fingers.
- Skip the butter on your jacket potato or sandwich.
- Swap to diet mixers in spirits.
- Choose fruit that's canned in fruit juice instead of syrup.
- Swap a glass of fruit juice for sugar-free cordial.

268. STAIRWAY TO HEAVEN

Next time you're faced with a flight of stairs, go up two at a time. It's an intense toning treatment that targets your thighs and bum. If you're new to exercise, start small and only go up two at a time for as long as it's comfortable.

269. SCRUB UP

Make your own zesty body scrub to wake your skin up every morning. Squeeze the juice of half an orange and 4 tbsp cornmeal into a bowl and mix into a paste. Apply all over your body and scrub in gently for two minutes. Rinse well, pat skin dry with a towel and moisturize.

270. SOYA SNACK

Tofu Kebabs. 132 calories.
Marinate 75 g (2¾ oz) of tofu cubes with 1 tbsp tomato puree, 1 tbsp light soy sauce, half a tbsp of sunflower oil, half a tbsp of honey and half a tbsp of wholegrain mustard for 10 minutes. Thread tofu cubes alternately on to skewers amongst chunks of red pepper, courgette and red onion. Grill for 10 minutes, turning frequently.

271. STAND LIKE A STAR

Body language is the icing on the cake when you're dressed up and feeling a million dollars. Don't let sloppy posture let down all that hard work. Stand tall, keep your chin up and look people in the eyes, it'll make you look and feel more confident.

272. VARNISHING ACT

Many manicurists shape the nail tip to match the natural shape at the base of your nail. Most women have squared off oval nail bases, so filing nails square at the end but with rounded edges suits most ladies. But if the base of your nails is square, don't round off your tips.

273. DRINK UP

Watermelons are full of antioxidants to help skin stay young. Whip up a non-alcoholic cocktail by cutting the flesh of a quarter of a melon into cubes and blending it until it's liquid (seeds might not be broken down but they taste good). Serve with mint leaves and ice.

274. STOMACH SHRINKER

Pineapple contains the enzyme bromelain that aids digestion and alleviates wind. But don't cook it or bromelain is destroyed. Instead sip a glass of pineapple juice with your breakfast.

275. BITE BY BITE

Studies show eating in a rush, watching television or holding a conversation stops you from keeping note of how much food you're tucking away. Eat slowly and in a peaceful atmosphere with no distractions so you're mindful of how much food you've eaten.

276. BLOW DRY

Avoid the dread of smudging freshly painted nails by blowing cold air on them with a hairdryer or dipping them into cool water. Both help to speed up the setting process and stop nails from smudging before they dry.

277. FAT ATTACK

Don't make the mistake of cutting back too much on fat which is essential for helping the body absorb vitamins A, D and E. Snacking on nuts and seeds is an easy way to get more healthy fats (see tip 138) and boosts the condition of skin and hair.

HAIR

278. TYING THE KNOT

For cute twists, spritz with hairspray and take 5 cm (2 in) sections of hair and twist tightly from the ends to the scalp. Keep twisting until each section coils back against your scalp like a knot, then secure it with crossed hairgrips for maximum hold. Let the ends stick out like spikes for an extra funky effect.

279. FIX FRIZZ

If you can't budge flyaway hairs or frizz, rub in a little leave in conditioner or moisturizer. It coats your hair shaft and gives hair extra weight to leave it flatter. Run fingers through hair but don't brush it and allow it to dry naturally.

280. HAIR TODAY, GONE TOMORROW

Hair loss can be triggered by stress, childbirth, bad health and over-styling. If you're loosing more locks than you're happy about, it's worth checking you don't have an iron deficiency. People who are losing a lot of hair are often low in Ferritin, a protein which helps the production of hair follicles and stores iron in the body. Foods with iron include:

- red meat
- liver
- fortified cereal
- eggs
- beans and pulses
- dried apricots, figs and dates
- watercress
- spinach

281. HAPPY ENDINGS

Split ends develop mostly in dry or brittle hair and can be caused by excessive dyeing or rigorous brushing. The only way to deal with them is to go for the chop. If you're growing your hair don't worry, it grows on average half an inch every month so it'll soon grow back. Have regular trims to prevent split ends travelling up the hair shaft.

282. FINE AND DANDY

Your scalp sheds small pieces of skin as part of the body's growth and regeneration process. But dandruff begins when small pieces of dead skin clump together if your scalp is too oily or too dry. The most effective solution is to buy a medicated anti-dandruff shampoo from your pharmacist.

283. COVER STORY

To make hair colour look natural it's wise to choose a tone that matches your skin type. As you get older you may be tempted to colour over grey hairs with bold colours but give it a miss. Skin lightens and loses its pigment with age so choose lighter tones to compliment your changing complexion.

284. ALL CHANGE

When considering what shade to colour hair it helps to first check out what tones suit your complexion, here's what works best:

- fair skin goes with blonde, auburn and brown tones, but avoid black.
- rosy cheeks suit ash blonde and brown hair, but avoid red.
- olive faces look good with deep auburn and mahogany shades, but avoid light colours.
- dark brown and black skin is suited to dark shades and rich highlights.

285. SMOOTH OPERATOR

Sleek hair down using products from around your home. Make yourself your own moisturizing spray by mixing three parts baby oil to three parts water in a spray bottle. After washing hair, blot off excess water with a towel, spray a little over ends and run fingers through it once it's dry.

286. ON THE STRAIGHT AND NARROW

Get a salon blow-dry at home. First, wash and condition hair and dry with a towel. When it's almost dry gather hair into sections and secure with clips. Starting with the bottom layers first, follow the brush down each section of your hair with your hairdryer until it's dry (keeping the dryer moving). Gradually work your way up the layers until all sections are straight. Finish with a blast of cool air (if your hairdryer has this function).

287. LATHER UP

Don't wash your hair more than once a day. Shampoos strip away natural oils that protect hair from damage and drying out. If you shampoo every day then choose a mild shampoo so your hair can keep enough natural oil to stay soft and glossy.

288. HOLD STILL

It can be a mission to get hair to stay put when it's pinned up for a special occasion or a big night out. The best product ever invented is hairspray for keeping styles in place and stray strands under control. You can choose between a variety of holds and it's great for adding shine

289. FAKE IT

Extensions can be made from either real or fake hair and in any length you prefer (but longer than 55 cm (22 in) can damage hair because the extra weight pulls on your scalp). There are several ways they're attached: strand-by-strand, in wefts (a track of several inches of hair already attached together at the top) and clip-on extensions. The key to making extensions look natural is to attach them in as small sections as you can, but preferably get the job done by a professional.

290. VA-VA-VOOM VOLUME

To lift roots, tip your head upside down once hair is 80 percent dry. Use a brush to lift hair gently away from the scalp and blast with your hairdryer until completely dry. Stand up straight and carefully make final touches to your hair without pressing on roots.

291. FUN IN THE SUN

If your hair is coloured, bleached or permed then it's extra vulnerable to sun damage. Protect it by washing hair in shampoos and conditioners containing sunscreens and wearing scarves or hats when you're on the beach or in the sun. Washing hair straight after swimming in pools or the sea also helps to limit the drying effects of chlorine and salt water so you have less bad hair days.

292. AU NATURALE

Putting hair up neatly can make you look too formal. Actress Sandra Bullock prefers to mess her hair up so it looks natural when she's got fancy frocks on for red carpet events. Tresses that aren't tampered with can play an outfit down perfectly.

293. COLOUR CRAZY

It's best to have permanent hair colour applied at a salon (see tip 323). That includes full head, highlights and lowlights. If you go ahead and do it yourself, bear in mind the further the colour from your natural shade then the sooner you'll have to touch up roots. (If you go wrong a bad dye job takes a long time to wash out.)

294. UP, UP AND AWAY

Do you know that tightly pulling hair back from your face is a sure way to draw attention to every wrinkle and flaw? Avoid ponytails or buns and opt for small slides or clips to hold stray hairs out of your eyes. Best of all, leave hair down around your face to soften features and hide blemishes.

295. STUBBLE TROUBLE

Get rid of unwanted body hair at home (after a visit to the chemist!) in the following ways:

- Shaving – razors remove the tip of your hair shaft that's grown out through the skin and lasts one to three days.
- Tweezing – pulls hair out from the root and lasts one to two weeks.
- Waxing – involves applying wax to target hairs, sticking a cloth to them and pulling them out from the roots and lasts two to four weeks.
- Depilatory creams – dissolves hair at the skin's surface and lasts one to three weeks.

296. BLACK BEAUTY

Afro hair contains less oil and fewer layers of cuticle per hair strand than other hair types, which means it feels more course and is vulnerable to damage. Make sure you only buy shampoos and conditioners with extra moisturizers and always wash hair very gently (to avoid pulling it when it's most fragile). Pat dry hair with a towel instead of rubbing it and never brush hair, use a wide-tooth comb or fingers instead. Condition it with a leave-in conditioner and limit blow-drying (as much as you can!).

297. FAST FIX

Oily looking roots come to most people sooner or later but if you don't have time to wash your hair or you want to fix the problem on the spot, then dab on dry shampoo powder which is available from good pharmacies. It zaps grease on the spot, but remember to wash it out well.

298. MAKING WAVES

For sexy, wavy hair all you have to do is set damp locks in small velcro rollers, roll them halfway up your hair, wait while they dry and then take them out and rake your fingers through. If you have thick hair choose medium rollers.

299. BRUSH UP

It's surprisingly relaxing if you brush your hair really slowly (and better still if you have someone else do it for you!). Use long, gentle strokes, starting at the front of your hairline where it meets your face and brush down to the nape of your neck. It goes over several calming acupressure points, relieving tension in your face, neck and shoulders.

300. EGGSTATIC

Eggs are a great source of protein, the body's building block for hair. Whip up your own conditioner using household products (so you save pennies for pampering elsewhere.) Beat an egg until it's frothy, add 1 tbsp baby oil and a cup of water and stir well. Apply to hair after shampooing and rinse out after ten minutes (or as long as you've got spare for super conditioning).

301. FACE FACTS

The following face shapes and hair styles go together:

- Oval faces suit most styles, but avoid spikes or piling hair up high as it adds volume to the top of your head, making your face look longer.
- Long faces are complimented by curls or waves, which add width and balance out your face.
- Round faces suit styles that lengthen the face like graduated layers. Avoid short, one length cuts.
- Square faces often include an angular jaw, so soften it by adding texture with short curls or long layers that begin below the chin.
- Heart faces tend to have pointed chins, but fringes that are swept to the side or sit on your eyebrows will draw attention to eyes instead.

302. SHINE ON

Rinse hair in cold water to maximize shine. Cool water makes hair cuticles contract and lie flat so your locks reflect more light and look more glossy. After rinsing pat hair dry with a towel (rubbing hair dry roughs up cuticles).

303. STOP STUBBLE

You can remove unwanted body hair permanently (and avoid shaving rash) and here's how:

- Laser hair removal, which uses a guided laser beam to kill hairs off so they can't grow back.
- Electrolysis, this involves a needle with an electric current being applied to hair follicles to destroy them.

Both need a course of treatment for best results.

304. SHAMPOO SAVVY

Perk up dull hair by spending more time rinsing out shampoo. The average dollop of shampoo needed to wash hair is the size of a tablespoon and should take four minutes of rinsing to get it all out.

305. PUMP UP THE VOLUME

Hair thickness is influenced by several factors including genetics, age, health problems and hair damage. But do you know how to check how thick your hair is to make sure you're using the right products? Here's how:

- Thin hair – when you pull your hair back in a ponytail it's 2 cm (1 in) or less thick and you can see some of your scalp after wetting hair.
- Medium hair – this is a good handful in thickness when gathered in a ponytail, the most common of all hair groups.
- Thick hair – hair is two fists in thickness when you scrape it back into a ponytail and it can be hard to manage or feel course.

306. WAXING LYRICAL

Make sure hair is long enough to wax (½ cm/¼ in at least) as wax needs enough hair to bind to otherwise it can't be pulled out at the root. Exfoliate legs with a body scrub the day before. Heat wax according to pack instructions and apply a small, thin layer one area at a time, going in the direction of hair growth. Before the wax cools apply a strip to the wax and remove quickly, peeling it in the opposite direction to the hair growth (it's less painful to keep the strip as close to the skin as possible).

307. FRESH START

When you're after a new hairstyle it pays to take a picture with you so the hairdresser can see exactly what you want. Build a good relationship with him or her so you're not worried to tell them exactly what you do and don't like. Questions to ask about a new hairstyle:

- How do I create it at home?
- Does it need any special products to maintain?
- How regularly do I need to visit the hair salon to keep it at its best?

308. HOT STUFF

Hair doesn't like high temperatures. Under the influence of hot air it becomes dry, frizzy, loses its gloss and can be hard to manage. If you need to dry your hair quickly, first massage a little blob of conditioner into hands and apply to ends. Then dry hair on your hairdryer's cool setting. If you don't have a cool button, make sure you use a heat protecting spray before blow-drying.

309. BOOZE IS BAD NEWS

Sorry wine lovers but alcohol is a diuretic so when you knock back your favourite tipple you're dehydrating your body. Excessive alcohol consumption also depletes nutrients like iron which can lead to hair loss.

310. THINK THIN

When you have thinning hair it's best to avoid centre partings which draws attention to your scalp and highlights thinning. Instead go for a tousled look or cut in layers to create volume, rather than keeping hair all one length which drags hair down, making it appear thinner.

311. MOISTURE IS A MUST

Leave-in conditioners help moisturize hair but they can weigh it down, so use sparingly. Rinse-out conditioners suit everyone and smooth out hair without making it lifeless. While hair masks are very effective deep conditioning treatments for coloured, bleached or permed hair and they should be left on for at least ten minutes (preferably under a warm towel).

312. BAD HAIR DAY

Serum is your best friend if you have frizzy hair. While hair is wet, rub a blob of serum the size of a grape between your palms and run it over the lengths and ends of your hair to seal and smooth hair cuticles down. Repeat a blob at a time so you don't overload hair and pin hair up so you can smooth hair down on bottom layers too.

313. BLONDE BOMBSHELL

Blonde hair comes in many different shades to suit every complexion. If you're fair then perhaps consider soft ash tones, if you're rosy go for deep ash shades and if you're dark or olive skinned you're best off with a medium beige blonde.

314. EYE FOR DETAIL
Choosing a new hair colour can be a tricky decision. A good tip is to choose a shade that compliments your eye colour:
- Dark brown eyes suit dark auburn, copper and coppery blonde hair.
- Light brown eyes look good with dark auburn or pastel blonde hair.
- Blue or light brown eyes work well with dark blonde hair.
- Hazel eyes suit golden brown and ash blonde hair.
- Green eyes compliment reddish blonde hair.

315. BUDGET BEAUTY
If you're broke then buy a cheap shampoo but invest in a good conditioner. Shampoo removes grime and oil from hair. But conditioner has lots of uses; it helps keep hair soft, shiny and easier to manage.

316. RESCUE REMEDY
If you're having a bad hair day, try tossing your tresses back into a ponytail with a pretty band or silk scarf. If your hair is short, introduce a new look with a headband or gently slide in a pretty hair clip.

317. CUT TO THE CHASE
If you go from hair that's all one length to a choppy look with layers then be prepared for the extra time it takes to style. Once hair is different lengths it becomes high maintenance. Consider your lifestyle and how much time you have before going for the chop.

318. TO DYE FOR
Different types of dye give you different looks as follows:
- Colour-enhancing shampoos give a tint to hair and boost your natural shade.
- Temporary colour products (like mousses) colour hair for up to three washes.
- Semi-permanent dyes wash out after six washes, but some can last for up to 20 washes.
- Permanent colour lasts two to three months.

319. CURLY WURLY
Mousse is the perfect product for creating waves and volume. Used mainly on fine or flat hair, it's great for blow-drying, finger-drying or scrunching to give roots lift.

320. SOFT TOUCH
The best way to condition hair after shampooing is to squeeze away excess water with your hands and then blot it with a towel (but don't rub or you can damage hair). Apply the recommended amount of conditioner that the product label suggests and work it through ends with a wide-tooth comb. Leave on as recommended, then rinse with cold water.

321. WAXWORK

With endless uses, hair wax can control frizz, slick back locks into sleek styles, define strands and build up shape. It's similar to gel but less wet on application and perfect for creating a choppy but casual look.

322. BOOST BOUNCE

Put body back into longer hair by gently pulling damp hair into a scrunchie or a big clip then shaking it out when it's dry (or you can spritz it with water if you aren't washing it).

323. HOME HAIRDRESSER

If you're dyeing your own hair, don't go for a dramatic colour change first time and leave permanent colour to a salon (see tip 293). Always read and follow pack instructions closely and do a skin and strand test at least 48 hours beforehand as allergic reactions can take a while to show up. Before starting smear Vaseline around the hairline so you don't dye skin and set an alarm clock to tell you when the time's up.

324. FAST FIX

If you're having a flat hair day or you've got a kinky fringe, dampen the roots in the problem area and lift hair with a brush until it's dry. Hey presto! Bad hair should be fixed within five minutes and no rollers required.

325. FRIZZ CONTROL

It might sound obvious, but consider a shorter style for summer if you have frizzy hair. Cropped hair is easier to control as well as being much cooler. But if you love your long hair then pile it on your head or tie it back to keep it under control.

326. HOLISTIC HAIR

Many countries have symbols printed on haircare products to show they're made from 100 percent organic ingredients. (Certifying organisations have also given the green light to skincare products too.) Opt for organic shampoos and conditioners which are kinder on damaged hair and prevent irritation to sensitive scalps.

327. FLOWER POWER

A-list ladies love a few petals in their hair when they're glamming up for big events. Silk flowers from arts and crafts stores look feminine and make a feature of hair without having to put in much effort. Hold them in place with criss-crossed grips.

328. ETHNIC HAIR

Afro-Caribbean hair needs extra TLC (see tip 296) and celebrity hair stylists recommend feeding hair with plenty of healthy fats. Eating oily fish such as mackerel, salmon, sardines and herrings or taking supplements with essential fatty acids (EFAs) helps improve the condition of hair from the inside out.

329. CLOSE SHAVE

Shaving can be a pain – literally! Men often have a problem with skin inflammation around the neck and face after shaving (folliculitis) and this condition is common in women as well. You can help limit irritation by shaving with a lubricating shaving cream to help the blade slide smoothly over skin. Then once you've finished shaving apply ice-cold aloe vera gel to close pores and cool skin (refrigerate the gel before using).

330. KNOT ATTACK

When hair gets tangled it can be a nightmare to manage (and not to mention reall painfull too!). Spritz a little leave-in conditioner and gently work a comb through knots, starting with the ends. Then shampoo and condition as normal. Never tackle tangles while the hair is wet as this is when it's most vulnerable and prone to breaking.

331. STRAIGHT TO THE POINT

For super straight hair, mist lengths with heat protection spray (see tip 308) and clip up the top layers. Using ceramic straightening irons, starting from the side of your lower layers, take a piece of hair about an inch wide and clamp the straighteners in close to your head without touching your scalp (or it could burn!). Slowly pull them down over the entire length of your hair and repeat throughout your lower layers. Unclip your top layer and do the same.

332. BLACK BEAUTY

Singer Mary J Blige adds colour to her dark afro hair by using clip in coloured extensions. They're an easy way of adding quick highlights to hair without having to keep colouring it, which can cause delicate afro hair to break.

333. STAND TO ATTENTION

If you spray hairspray onto a tissue and run it over your hair you can wave goodbye to static. But try to avoid using your hands, which makes hair more greasy. If you've got fabric conditioner sheets that are designed for tumble dryers, they're just as good and they leave a lovely smell.

334. WATER WORKS WONDERS

If your hair loses its shape throughout the day, just mist it lightly with a little water. It reactivates the styling products in your hair, so you can reshape or tidy up without needing lots of products to hand.

335. ROOT CAUSE

Growing out colour or bleach can make hair look scruffy (unless you're going for a boho look!) so consider having a semi-permanent colour all over. It evens up colour and conditions hair for that tricky in-between phase. Visit a hair salon for best results.

336. FAKE IT

If you've lost your hair there are fantastic quality wigs on the market. In fact some celebrities wear them to give their own hair a break from styling. Wigs are made from synthetic hair, real hair or a combination of both. Synthetic wigs look real but feel fake and you can't style them. So choose wigs made from real hair or a combination of both to look your best.

337. SHORT STORY
Ways to make the most out of short hair:
- Use styling wax on damp hair to add texture and definition.
- Use shine spray for a glossy sheen.
- Trim hair every six weeks, growth shows up faster on short styles.
- Wash hair frequently to prevent greasy roots.

338. NEED A LIFT?
If you haven't got time to blow-dry your hair, supermodel Helena Christensen swears by towel-drying hair before scooping it up into a bun for the rest of the day and letting it air dry. When you let your hair down it will be naturally wavy with lots of volume.

339. CUTTING EDGE
Avoid crossing your legs when you're getting your hair cut. Sitting pretty with one leg over the other will alter your posture and leave you with an uneven cut. Sit up straight with your legs together for a better result.

340. PLASTER DISASTER
Avoid having to stick plasters all over your shaving cuts. Instead, shave during a bath or shower – it's less hassle and razor blades glide better and last longer. Use a shaving gel or cream and go lightly over areas that are less fleshy like ankles, knees and shins to avoid cuts.

341. NICE KNOT

Gather hair into a neat ponytail at the nape of your neck and secure with a band. Lightly backcomb your ponytail to give it some body. Then take three-quarters of the ponytail and poke part of it through the band again to create a loop. Twist the remaining ends of your hair around the band and loop to cover the band. Secure everything in place with grips and hairspray.

342. ROOT CAUSE

There are fantastic root touch-up kits on the market to cover grey hair or root regrowth for that awkward stage in between hair colouring appointments. Kits feature easy to use brushes so you can dab colour on problem areas like your hairline or centre parting.

STYLE

343. FIGURE IT OUT

Work out your body shape and dress to flatter your figure. Here's how:

- Pear shapes – you store fat mostly on hips, bums and thighs. Dark coloured skirts and trousers will slim down your bottom half to balance up proportions.
- Apple shapes – your weight is usually found around your middle, while your arms and legs are pretty slim. Tops that are snug under the chest but skim your stomach will flatter a fuller tummy.
- Hourglass – you have a womanly figure with big boobs, small waist and big hips. Tops and jackets that nip you in at the waist will make the most of your slim stomach.

344. TANTALISING

Show off a tan by wearing white at every opportunity. It's the best colour because it contrasts with brown skin and accentuates darker skin tones so you end up looking more brown. But that's not all…white reflects light towards your skin which helps you look young again!

345. LEARN YOUR LINES

Only wear horizontal stripes if you're flat-chested and want to look more curvy. Stripes that run across, rather than down, make you look wider so only the slender can get away with it. If you're a fan of stripes but you're worried about looking bigger, buy striped accessories instead.

346. PERFECT PINS

Cropped trousers or anything that ends above the ankle make legs appear shorter. Create the illusion of longer legs with high-waisted trousers or skirts to make your bottom half appear longer. Trousers should be flared and long enough to just about skim the floor and cover any shoe no matter how high. You can push the look to the max with a three-quarter length jacket or a dress worn over trousers to disguise short legs.

347. BOSOM BUDDIES

If you're a woman reading this then the chances are seven out of ten of you aren't wearing a correctly fitted bra according to research. Most department stores offer a free fitting service and you'll be amazed how different tops look when you wear the right size bra. Boobs will be lifted, accentuating your waist, and posture will be improved by holding your shoulders back.

348. BITS AND BOBS

Actresses Sienna Miller and Sarah Jessica Parker like to accessorize clothes with costume jewellery to stamp their own style on an outfit. Buying quirky bags, belts or shoes is a great way of expressing your personality. Mix and match them with your regular clothes to create different looks without breaking the bank.

349. CLUELESS ABOUT COLOUR?

Open your wardrobe and pick out clothes in the colours you wear most often. Make a pile of the different colour groups, then one colour at a time, put each item up against your face in front of a mirror in a good light. Now study your face. Note which colours bring out flaws like dark circles under your eyes or red cheeks. These are your wrong colours. What shades brighten up your eyes and make your skin look at its best? This is the colour category you should dress in.

350. BOOBY PRIZE

If you have a large bust then opt for a V-neck to break up the big expanse of chest area on your body. It'll make boobs look in better proportion. Try to avoid roll necks, no matter how much you like them, they're high cut and make large chests appear even bigger. Oversized tops don't fix the problem either, they'll make you look as big as a house.

351. OFF THE CUFF

If you've got sturdy wrists you can carry off chunky bracelets and watches but if you're small boned then go for delicate bracelets. Charity shops are brilliant sources for unusual pieces and can give you the perfect finishing touch to a special outfit.

352. LEGGY LESSON

You can't go wrong with black opaque tights to make legs look longer and slimmer. Patterns like narrow weave fishnets and vertical stripes are also flattering for shapely legs, but go for dark colours so legs appear slender.

353. BELT UP

Wearing the right belt is down to how wide it is and where you wear it. If you have a short upper body then be careful with chunky belts because they cover what waist you have, making you look wider. Be cunning about where you place your belt too. Is it more flattering worn low slung on your hips or high up and cinching your waist? People's eyes will go to wherever you choose, so think before you buckle up.

354. GIVE BULGES THE BOOT

Boots can help heavy legs look better under skirts as long as you avoid mid-calf and ankle lengths, which make chunky legs look even bigger. Knee boots with a heel will elongate legs perfectly so you can wave goodbye to podgy pins. Always avoid baggy styles which bulk out legs.

355. KNICKERS IN A TWIST

Figure-fixing underwear has come a long way since old-fashioned corsets. Sales are soaring for support knickers and shorts, widely available in department stores and good underwear shops. When you wear a pair they take inches off bums, tums and hips instantly, making them fantastic for wearing under dresses on special occasions.

356. PAIN IN THE NECK

If you have a short neck, double chin or big breasts, then necklaces should be one of the lesser items in your accessory stash. Always choose necklaces that are delicate and simple in design if you're neck isn't you're best feature. If on the other hand you've got a long neck, you'll suit most necklaces from chokers to dangly beads.

357. WELL-HEELED

Singer Gwen Stefani slips on a pair of stilettos when she wants to make an outfit look sexy. Wearing high heels changes the way you stand because they throw your weight forward on to your toes, causing your back to arch slightly and your bum to stick out (that's why men like these shoes!). It's also harder work to stand and walk so your tummy muscles get pulled in as you try harder to balance.

358. BOOST YOUR ASSETS

Dress to suit your shape and make the most of your best bits. Fashion that flatters your body is a basic rule of dressing no matter what trends are in vogue. Clothes that skim over your trouble spots can lift your self-esteem. Why would you draw attention to bits you feel bad about? It will only make you focus on your faults and get you down.

359. SHOP SAVVY

Don't chuck money down the drain on designer clothes because you can look just as good shopping on the High Street. Pay attention to the cut of an outfit and not the label on the back (seriously, money doesn't buy you style). As long as you have clothes that fit your body properly then you'll always look great. Shop around until you find the retailers that cut best for your shape.

360. BEST FOOT FORWARD

Grab some pointy shoes if you have petite feet and feel self conscious at big events or in important photos. They add the illusion of length and make your feet look more in proportion to the rest of your body. Flats or heels with points will both give a flattering effect.

361. WAIST DISPOSAL

Hide a big belly and create the illusion of a nipped in waist with some sly shopping. Bin baggy clothing which hide curves and makes you look even bigger. Put tailored jackets at the top of your list, they naturally pull you in at the waist and flare out over hips. Invest in tops with a bit of boning for that elusive hourglass figure. Wrap tops are great at creating curves in a flattering way, particularly when they tie at the side of the waist.

362. GET A HEAD START

Hats can provide a finishing touch to outfits and save time fussing over hair. But certain styles suit certain shape faces. High foreheads go well with beanies and low foreheads look best with high-crowned hats. But if you want to flatter a fuller face then wear a wide brim to be in proportion with your head and shoulders.

363. SADDLE BAGS

Excess fat around hips is common for millions of women, but it affects men too when they're very overweight. Avoid bottoms that are low-cut or tight unless you want to create a 'muffin top' appearance. Instead, balance out your shape with slash neck tops which widen the neckline in proportion with big hips. Choose A-line skirts, which glide over bumps and swap tapered trousers for flares to flatter hips.

364. RING IN THE CHANGES

There's a ring out there to suit everyone. If you have small-boned fingers stay away from bold designs and big shapes and choose delicate antique pieces or styles with detailed designs. But for chunky hands and fingers go for big sizes and really bold designs. When you find a ring you love you can make a feature of it on your hand, rather than wearing loads of rings and cluttering fingers up.

365. BACK TO BLACK

Matching a black leather bag with black shoes is good for formal events, but it isn't the only way to match your accessories. Go for a modern look and look for muted browns, plums and greens which will work with most colours and are more versatile than black. It's not vital that shoes match your bag exactly either (so you can breathe a sigh of relief!). Experiment to see what works.

366. THIGH AND MIGHTY

Big legs can make wearing trousers a nightmare. For a quick fix buy some underwear support shorts which are available from department stores and good lingerie shops. Made from extra-thick lycra, they redistribute flesh around the bum and thigh area more evenly and pull you in, giving the appearance of being thinner.

367. ELEGANT EARS

Choose earrings to suit your face shape. Long faces look good in chandelier-shaped earrings and can carry off studs. Round faces suit slightly dangly styles which skim the face. Always choose colours to compliment your outfit.

368. BACK TO BASICS

Do you have extra flesh that spills over your bra at the back? You can get rid of back bulges quickly by wearing a bra with wide straps. It distributes the pulling power over a wider area and stops bras pinching flesh and causing those annoying bumps of back fat.

369. RED ALERT

Red is difficult to wear so it's important to test out which tones match your complexion. If you're quite red faced or a fake tan devotee it will bring out the lobster in you. Instead red looks best against pale white or black skin and the trick is to wear it with other hot coloured accessories like fuschia and orange. The most common mistake is to team red with black or white, which is overpowering.

370. LEG OVER

Even slim women have to put up with big calves and ankles which make legs look out of proportion. If this is you then avoid skirts that end mid-calf and go for A-line skirts instead because the wider the hem, the slimmer the ankle. Swap cropped trousers for long flares, which wont grip to calves, and wear high heels underneath to lengthen legs.

371. JELLY BELLY

If you're bored of hiding a bulging tummy under jackets for work then look for tops with shirt tail hems. They're cut to curve over the front of tummies while lifting at the side to reveal a slimmer hip bone. Ruched tops also dress up an outfit and make it hard for people to see the difference between gathers in the fabric and your spare tyres. Always choose low-cut skirts and trousers, which cut across the stomach and make it look half the size.

372. SHAPE UP

Slipping on a pair of flattering shoes can reshape your body and legs. You've probably heard it before, but heels really do lengthen your figure and make you look slimmer as long as you get the right heel. Delicate kitten-heels make calves appear chunkier. While ankle straps draw attention to big ankles. If you have big legs your best bet is wearing wedges, they're heavy enough to balance out the most sturdy calves or ankles.

373. GREY IS GREAT

Black doesn't suit everyone, but grey is a good alternative and can look very sophisticated. Grey is mostly a daytime colour but it's fairly versatile and silvery shades work well at night. If you have red hair, hazel eyes and freckly skin then it's not the colour for you, but blue eyes and black hair really bring this shade to life.

374. GET PERSONAL

You know how Hollywood stars have personal shoppers? Well did you know they're available to you for free? Many High Street stores offer this service free to its customers, or you can treat yourself to a personal stylist. It's an easy way to get a good makeover if you're bored of your look.

375. BINGO WINGS

Flatter flabby arms by wearing three-quarter length sleeves. They expose the slimmest part of the arm, your wrist, and draw the eye lower down the arm. For extra confidence cover up with cardigans, shrugs, boleros, shawls or jackets.

376. BUTTON IT

Small details on clothes can make a big difference. Choose outfits with chunky or oversized buttons if you have a big frame. Plus when you're wearing jackets and cardigans, only do the top few buttons up. Letting the rest of the cardigan hang open will skim curves beautifully.

377. WRAP UP

Coats can hide a lot of problem areas or they can emphasize them. So don't get it wrong because they make the first impression when you walk in a room. Ladies should avoid double-breasted styles, which make you look broad. Flattering styles include belted coats to emphasize waists or knee-lengths styles to cover bums and tums.

378. PRINTWORKS

Every fashion season brings with it a new set of prints but a general rule, no matter what the trend, is that big prints are for big bodies and fine prints for petites. Large prints are more slimming than little prints because there's less repetition across the body and they give the optical illusion that the wearer is slimmer.

379. MATERIAL GIRL

Why is it that some clothes look lovely on the hanger but when you put them on it's a disaster? It's down to the fabric. Clingy materials such as lycra and jersey stick to your biggest areas like stomachs and bums. While woven fabrics such as cotton or silk give you more room to disguise bits that you don't like.

380. COLOUR IS CRUCIAL

People who are huge fans of wearing black should always include one piece of colour and put it somewhere you want to draw attention. It might be red shoes with a black suit or a pink handbag with a black dress. Colour can work for everyone by drawing people's eyes to your best features.

381. TUMMY TAMER

Wide waistbands are the best friend of anyone with a wobbly waistline because they provide more support and hold you in a treat. Chunky bands are more in proportion with a larger tummy, whereas small waistbands only make the rest of your tummy look even bigger.

382. JEANIUS

Jeans are one of the most versatile items of clothing in everyone's wardrobe but make sure you get the right pair for your shape. High-waisted jeans emphasize bums and tums so if you're pear shaped avoid them and choose hipsters instead. The cut of the leg is just as vital. Tapered jeans only flatter slim people where as boot cut styles and flares suit most shapes and the thicker the denim the better if you need holding in.

383. SMART MOVE

Fitted jackets are flattering for all shapes and fantastic for dressing down with jeans or glamming up with heels and sparkly accessories. If you're worried about looking too smart, shop around for a jacket in a bold colour or funky fabric for a casual feel.

384. IT'S A WRAP
Scarves are really handy accessories for men and women. They add glamour, lend colour to your face, focus the eye away from your body and can express your personality. Buy a variety of print, colours and textures and you'll never be stuck for making an outfit special.

385. BEACH BABE
Curvy girls can feel confident about their tummies on the beach by swapping bikinis for tankinis. The vest top in a tankini set gives good bust and tummy support and covers bellies completely. They're much more modern than old-fashioned one piece swimsuits and you can always roll the top up when nobody's watching and get a tanned tummy.

386. TALL STORY
If you want to add a bit of height then go for vertical stripes and lines. Whether you choose pleats, patterns or plain old stripey prints, they'll all elongate your body and make you appear slimmer and trimmer. Subtle stripes include pinstripes, cord and ribbed sweaters.

387. GLITZ AND GLAMOUR
When you're dressing for a special event it can be tempting to throw together lots of glitzy pieces at once. But be careful you don't end up looking more sparkly than a Christmas tree. Pick one item of clothing that's striking and keep everything else understated or simple.

388. CATWALK CREATIONS
You don't need a big budget to keep up with catwalk trends. Rediscover the benefits of the high street, which is now super fast at creating outfits that are close to the catwalk originals and at a fraction of the price.

389. BOOB BOOSTER
Here's how to cheat if you're flat-chested:
- Push-up bras are a woman's best friend. They lift and enlarge breasts gently to give you a fantastic fullness and pert shape.
- Padded bras can work miracles. The extra wadding can boost boobs by a cup size.
- Balcony bras subtly enhance small boobs with a low-cut design, while some styles include extra padding.
- Stick-in pads are popular with celebrities for boosting their cup size. Commonly called chicken fillets, due to their size and shape, you can find them in good underwear stores.

390. COLOUR COMBO
When mixing coloured clothes don't wear three or more completely different coloured items of clothing at once, unless you want to look like a clown! Black, white and grey go with any colours. But keep bright colours to your top half and darks to your bottom for a slimming effect.

391. COPY CAT

Singer and actress Jennifer Lopez takes inspiration from the late Marilyn Monroe and Jacqueline Onassis when it comes to fashion. Don't be afraid to pay homage to your favourite celebrity's clothes or be inspired by people in the street. If something catches your eye on a stranger, stop and ask them where they got it. You'll save hours trying to look for something similar in the shops and they'll be flattered!

392. STOCKING FILLER

Avoid hold-ups slipping down by making sure the skin around your thighs is dry. Any grease or moisture, such as residue left over from body moisturizer will prevent the band along the top of stockings from sticking properly to skin.

393. NOTHING TO LOOSE

Teaming a bulky sweater with thick, wide trousers will make you look like you've gained weight. At the other extreme if you combine a figure hugging skirt with a tight T-shirt you could be showing off too much shape for formal occasions. A good rule to follow is to remember that loose clothes on your top half should be combined with slim clothes on the bottom, and vice versa. For example, a fitted shirt looks fabulous with flared trousers and a pair of skinny jeans go wonderfully with a loose top.

394. RECLYCLE AND REVAMP

You don't have to rush out and buy a whole new wardrobe after reading this book. You can work with what you've got. The most important aspect of dressing is that your clothes fit your body. Alter clothes so they fit you better and look more fashionable (pay to get them altered for a top notch job or if you're useless with a needle and cotton).

395. A CUT ABOVE

In terms of style and sophistication, a black dress for women or a black suit for men is hard to beat. If there's one outfit you should have in your wardrobe it's a little black dress (LBD). A well-made, classically cut dress will never go out of fashion and it can be won in so many different ways that it's worth its weight in gold.

396. STOP SAGGING

All ladies should get a sports bra for exercising. The extra comfort and support will prevent damage to delicate breasts, not to mention the pain of straining and stretching such a delicate area.

397. BOBBLY BITS

If your outfit picks up fluff, hair or other bits and bobs throughout the day (which shows up straight away on black), then make yourself an emergency fluff remover by cutting off a small piece of sticky tape and lightly pressing it over clothes.

398. HOLE IN ONE

If you get a ladder in your tights, pop socks or stockings then grab some clear nail varnish and dab a little lightly around the edges. It will instantly stop it getting bigger until you can get yourself a new pair.

399. ADDED EXTRAS

Accessories can make or break an outfit. If you've got a few pieces on, how do you know if you're wearing too much? Stand in front of a mirror, close your eyes, then open them, what's the first accessory that caught your eye? Take it off.

400. BEST FOOT FORWARD

Gorgeous shoes may look beautiful but if they hurt your feet then you'll walk like you're decades older. They'll also cause a huge variety of problems with feet, knees and backs. When buying fancy footwear such as stilettos, always try them on at the end of the day when your feet are most tired and swollen.

401. STICK OR TWIST?

Never get caught out with sticky price labels still attached to clothes or shoes. If you have trouble peeling labels off, give them a blast with a hairdryer to heat up the adhesive. They'll peel away a lot easier.

402. CLASSIC CLOTHING

Stand out from the crowd with vintage clothing. Celebrity stylists hunt through markets, secondhand clothing stores and the Internet for one-off pieces to dress their clients in. You can mix and match old clothes with modern basics to achieve a variety of looks.

403. V FOR VICTORY

Celebrity stylists will tell you that V-necks hide a multitude of sins. Create the illusion of a longer neck, smaller boobs or distract attention from a podgy tummy with V-neck sweaters. They work well with jeans for a casual look or black trousers when you need to look smart.

404. RAISE YOUR GLASSES

Choose specs and shades to suit your face shape, here's how:

- If you have a round face go for square-shaped lenses which create a more angular look.
- Oval and heart faces are complemented by frames which slant towards the temples to make a feature of the eye area.
- Square faces should buy frames that are straight along the top and curved underneath to add roundness in the right places.

405. STYLE WITH STAYING POWER

When you're going to an all-day event like a wedding your best approach is to opt for layering and that way you can dress an outfit up or down. A good option is wearing a dress with a jacket or sequined shrug that can be took off in the evening for a casual look.

406. PUMP IT UP

You might think ballet pumps are a sensible option, but flats with no cushioning under your foot cause bad posture and aching feet. Slip in an insole with heel support to straighten up posture. You'll find them in good pharmacies or visit a podiatrist for specially moulded alternatives.

407. UNDERCOVER STORY

Look your best in your evening dress by choosing the right support underwear to suit your shape (see tip 343), here's how:

- Hourglass shapes should wear support knickers to control hips and a basque or corset to show off a slim waist.
- Apples need high-waisted support shorts to flatten their tummy and a push up bra to enlarge breasts and draw eyes elsewhere.
- Pear body shapes should go for control knickers to slim hips and a push up bra to balance out body shape.

408. BLOCKBUSTER

It really cheers up a dull complexion to wear bright colours and it's a trend that suits everyone. Wearing block colours looks good as long as you team it up with dark colours such as black tights under a bright dress or navy jeans with a coloured jacket. For a more subtle look go for bold coloured accessories.

409. SWEATER STYLE

Bulky knits might keep you warm but the chunkier the knit, the chunkier you'll look. Avoid making a fashion faux pas by adding a big belt around your waist to show off your curves if you're wearing thick jumpers. But better still, opt for fine knits as a rule.

410. BIKINI BODY

Choose swimwear to flatter your figure:

- Flat chests are best suited to bikini tops with padding, frills or horizontal stripes which make chests look bigger. Underwired bikini tops help create more shape too.
- Big bums look great in dark coloured bikini briefs and prints on top. Briefs with wrap skirts attached will flatter lumps and bumps perfectly.
- Big breasts look good in V-neck swimsuits which lengthen the upper body and draw eyes downwards. Choose thick shoulder straps in proportion with bust size.
- Big bellies are well hidden under a tankini (see tip 385), vest tops cover a wobbly waist while built in cup support boosts boobs.

411. LESS IS MORE

Matching earrings and necklace sets are overpowering if they're worn together. When dressing up for big events, Hollywood actress Salma Hayek says she only wears a necklace if earrings are small and simple. Then if she's got big earrings on, she ditches necklaces altogether.

412. GOLDEN GODDESS

Everyone can look great on the beach with the help of a sarong. It can be wrapped around your body and neck as a sundress or tied around your waist to cover up big bums, tums or thighs. Add some wedge sandals instead of flip flops for a slim silhouette.

413. DRESSED TO IMPRESS

Choose dresses to flatter your body shape, here's how:
- Hourglass figures suit dresses fitted tightly at the waist or designs with a bodice and boning (or save money and nip in your waist with a thick belt).
- Apple shapes should try empire line dresses which gather under the bust and flair over tummies.
- Pears should go for a style that balances out their top and bottom half. Halternecks broaden shoulders inline with big hips.

414. BUDGET BUYS

It pays to invest in a few pieces of expensive, well made pieces of clothing and save on cheaper items elsewhere. Splurge on: suits, coats, shoes and bags. Save on: T-shirts, shirts, sweaters, summer dresses, scarves and belts.

415. SMARTY PANTS

Choose briefs to match your outfit:

- Flesh coloured knickers are great for blending in with your skin tone under see through clothes.
- G-strings are fab for clingy outfits that give you a visible panty line (VPL).
- Boy shorts give you a smooth line under figure hugging skirts and dresses.
- Hipsters are cut low enough to stay hidden under low-slung jeans and trousers.

416. MIX IT UP

Silver and gold jewellery shouldn't be worn together if you're a classic dresser or you like to stick to traditional styles. But if you're after an edgy look then mixing metals can work well.

417. HOLE IN ONE

Never ever worry about looking big on the beach again. Before you put your towel down, hollow out a dent in the sand where your bum will rest. Then when you lie down you'll sink into the sand and look super slim.

418. MINIMISE MARKS

Avoid getting white marks on black tops or dresses by using special antiperspirants that are designed not to leave residue, available from pharmacies. If you do get marks, gently sponge off with warm water.

419. SIMPLE STYLE

Actress Teri Hatcher stocks her wardrobe with classic styles that don't date in a hurry but suit her figure. She reckons she can dress up basic clothes with glamorous accessories to get the prefect look for every occasion without shopping for new outfits.

420. PANTYHOSE POSE

Like a girdle for legs, body-contouring tights are fab for eliminating bulges in legs or under skirts and dresses. As well as smoothing lumpy bits, they're particularly good for giving you an extra layer of support if you've got a big tummy. Look out for them in good pharmacies and department stores.

421. PERFECT PACKING

Roll your clothes instead of folding them, it reduces the amount of creases and takes up less space. Delicate dresses should be rolled with a layer of bubble wrap (or a towel) to prevent little creases. Pack socks and tights inside shoes to help them keep their shape.

422. BOTTOMS UP

Perk up a saggy bum instantly by investing in padded knickers. All good department stores and underwear specialists stock them and they give you a great rounded shape. To increase the size of your derriere even more, choose trousers or jeans with details over the bum area too.

FRAGRANCE

423. SMELL OF SUCCESS

The vanilla bean is great for hiding odours, especially cooking smells and studies suggest smelling it can help fight cravings for sweet food. Drop 1–2 tsp of natural vanilla extract in a small cup anywhere around the home (or put it in the kitchen if you're likely to raid the fridge).

424. EVERYDAY ESSENTIALS

Derived from plants, essential oils are used in aromatherapy to alter the state of your body and mind. When you use essential oils on your skin always dilute them in a vegetable carrier oil such as sunflower or almond oil. Use approximately six drops of essential oil to 25 ml (5 tsp) of carrier oil. Putting six drops of essential oil in a bath or a few drops on a handkerchief is enough to get the benefit of each oil's properties.

425. FRESHEN UP

Did you know hair companies have started doing fragrances for hair? Visit a good pharmacy and test out smells until you find your favourite. Then spritz a little over your hair to cover smells picked up by smoking, cooking or plain old hair grease if you've not had time to wash your hair.

426. FRAGRANCE FABRICS

If you have sensitive skin you can spritz your perfume over fabrics so you still smell nice. Avoid spraying scents on the outside of your clothes because some formulations may stain. Instead add a little to the inner hem or lining of your clothes and as your body temperature rises, so will the fragrance.

427. GO POTTY

Plants can scent your home and act as natural air filters at the same time. Houseplants like English ivy and poinsettas are particularly helpful at keeping air toxin-free and removing chemicals released by furniture and carpets, stopping them circulating around your home.

428. SCENTSATIONAL

Try a new perfume. First work out which fragrance group most applies to you, then choose a new scent:

- Feminine – lily of the valley, orange blossom, jasmine, rose
- Romantic – vanilla, amber
- Fougere (meaning 'Fern' in French) – lavender, rosemary, mint, geranium
- Chypre (meaning 'Cyprus' in French) – bergamot, lemon, grapefruit

429. SOFTER SKIN

In the summer it's beneficial for skin to use a scented body oil or lotion instead of perfume. Take your time massaging it into skin before dressing. Once it's soaked in you'll enjoy super soft skin and smell good enough to eat.

430. SPOIL YOURSELF WITH OIL

Essential oils have different physical and mental effects:

- Camomile – reduces anxiety and aids relaxation.
- Eucalyptus – revives the body and clears the head.
- Jasmine – boost moods and reduces anxiety.
- Lavender – soothes skin and aids relaxation.
- Lemon – enhances concentration and is a good pick-me-up.
- Peppermint – helps digestion.
- Rosemary – fights off fatigue and stimulates body and mind.

431. FINGER ON THE PULSE
Ever wondered why experts recommend spraying perfume on the inside of your wrists? Placing scents on pulse points (behind ears and knees and on temples and wrists) is where your body gives off more heat. So it acts like a mini fragrance pump.

432. LOVE LEMON
Pack lemongrass oil when you're off on holiday. You can dab a few drops on some tissue to revive you when you're jetlagged and it's also a handy natural deodorant in hot climates.

433. SPRAY AWAY
Choose the right strength of fragrance:
- Perfume (also known as parfum) is more concentrated than other types of fragrance, so a little goes a long way, but it's more expensive.
- Eau de Toilette is the most popular fragrance sold because it's cheaper than perfume but less concentrated.
- Cologne is the name given to scents for men that are citrus-based and generally much softer than perfume or Eau de Toilette.

434. HOME SWEET HOME
Add a few drops of your favourite essential oil or perfume to a cotton wool ball and place it in your vacuum cleaner bag. Lemon and pine scents are a great choice for freshening up rooms. You can also add five drops of essential oil to fabric conditioner to cover up smelly clothes. Both will scent the house beautifully while clothes dry and you'll smell fresh all day long.

435. 40 WINKS
Lavender is renowned for its relaxation properties and helping people get to sleep. Add a few drops of essential oil to a tissue and slip it in your pillowcase or place a handful of dried lavender in a pretty container next to your bed to lull you into a deep sleep.

436. MINT CONDITION
When you're feeling tired, mint is wonderfully refreshing and gives you a lift when you're feeling low. Suck on mints and add a handful of mint leaf stems to a vase of flowers (but pick flowers that aren't strongly scented).

437. PLAY YOUR CARDS RIGHT

If you find a new perfume you like, take a few test cards away with you first. When you get home, wait a few hours and see if you still like it. Some perfumes smell great at first but they completely change once they've been on for hours.

438. NO SWEAT

Perspiring is normal and natural, it's what your body does to maintain the right temperature. Did you know sweat itself doesn't smell bad? It's the bacteria that feeds on sweat that makes such a whiff. Wash regularly and avoid synthetic fabrics, which trap heat. Plus use a deodorant (which masks the smell) or an anti-perspirant (which limits sweating).

439. AROMA ZONE

Combine beautiful smells with a relaxing atmosphere and splash out on some scented candles. Make sure they're made using essential oils rather than synthetic perfume, so you can enjoy the benefits of aromatherapy (see tip 430), while you chill out in the candlelight. Never leave a naked flame unattended.

440. BATH BLEND

Wake yourself up by adding five drops of sandalwood, three drops of sweet orange and one drop of ginger essential oil to your bath water. For a relaxing bath add five drops of lavender oil, two drops of chamomile and two drops of clary sage instead.

441. LOVE POTION

If you want to attract the opposite sex then wear perfume containing cedarwood, ylng ylang, sandalwood or cardamom. They're all aphrodisiac fragrances which will get people drooling once a waft comes their way.

442. FANCY FOOTWORK

Change your shoes every day and wear socks made from natural fibres such as cotton to help skin breathe and limit foot odour. Use a refreshing foot spray to cool feet down during in summer, they're made to keep you smelling sweet.

WELL-BEING

443. CUDDLE UP

Giving someone you love a hug can lower blood pressure and release the feel good chemical oxytocin which helps you relax. Snuggling up also cuts levels of cortisol, a stress hormone which lowers your immune system and stores fat around your tummy.

444. STRESS BUSTER

Find a quiet room, lie down on your back, get comfortable and close your eyes. Clench your toes and release them a few times, then let them relax. Move up your body in the same fashion - tensing and releasing your legs, then hips, bum, stomach, hands, arms, chest, neck and finally your face. You'll be super floppy at the end of it and totally tension-free.

445. BRAIN FOOD

Serotonin is one of the most important brain chemicals for regulating moods. Your body makes it from the amino acid tryptophan, found naturally in the these foods:

- turkey
- chicken
- fish
- cottage cheese
- bananas
- eggs
- nuts
- avocados
- milk
- cheese
- beans

446. HAVE A GIGGLE

Laughter is the best medicine. Studies suggest it helps with everything from boosting the immune system to feeling less pain. Find something to raise a smile every day (it doesn't matter how silly). Small things like reading a comic, going to a comedy club with friends or playing children's game can be enough to make you chuckle.

447. TIME OUT

It can be tempting to work late when you've got mountains of work. But leave your workload behind and use an answer machine to screen calls once you've clocked off. Treating activities with family and friends like work commitments or meetings you can't miss will help you keep a healthy balance of work and play.

448. BEAUTY BOOST

When you're tired, depressed or feeling low it's useful to make the effort to do your hair, paint your nails or apply some make-up. It might seem like too much effort to start with but you'll feel better about yourself when you know you're looking good. Hollywood actress Kate Winslet always makes sure she puts on a little make-up every morning.

449. SIP AND SNOOZE

Swap caffeinated drinks for herbal teas. Caffeine acts like a stimulant and stays in the body hours after you've had it. It can leave you wide-awake and really frustrated when you want to sleep. Choose chamomile tea before bed, it's a gentle sedative as well as helping your digestion if you've eaten late. You can find caffeine in:

- tea
- coffee
- energy drinks
- cola
- chocolate

450. WRITE ON

Stockpile all your happy memories by keeping photos, videos and notes so you can relive special moments when you're feeling tired or low. Revisiting cherished memories gives you a positive focus and distracts you from negative thoughts during difficult times.

451. SMALL TALK

Offering a compliment to someone makes you feel just as good as the person on the receiving end. It makes you feel nice because you know you've done a good thing and it doesn't hurt that it'll earn you friends!

452. FEET TREAT

Any podiatrist will tell you good health begins with good feet. It seems obvious, but wearing comfortable shoes will help you feel relaxed, relieve pressure from aching feet and help with posture problems. Women who love heels higher than 2.5 cm (1 in) should only wear them on special occasions and do all their walking in trainers.

453. HANDS-ON APPROACH

Get somebody to give you a quick massage or better still splash out and get a professional to do it! Studies show it boosts blood flow to the skin, drains excess fluid to reduce puffiness and nourishes skin cells. So skin looks plumper, firmer and brighter.

454. HAPPY DAYS

Seeing the brighter side of life not only makes you feel better about yourself but it improves health problems. If you're a 'glass half-full' person you're likely to be happy with your life and less likely to let stress get to you. Research shows a positive attitude gives you lower blood pressure.

455. ACT LIKE AN ANGEL

Make small gestures to help others. It doesn't mean you have to run a marathon for charity, but little things like helping mums up steps with pushchairs, holding doors open for a stranger or inviting your neighbour in for a cup of tea can all make you feel good about yourself.

456. GO MAD FOR 10 MINUTES

Studies show you're happier when you're feeling energetic. Give yourself a quick shot of energy with a brisk ten minute walk outside in sunlight if possible (it really does work, even if you feel tired at the start). If you'd prefer to stay in, listen to some upbeat music and have a boogie around the house.

457. FURRY FRIENDS
Studies show having a pet makes you happier and healthier. Keeping animals helps with stress management and lowers blood pressure. Having a dog is particularly good for you because it encourages owners to get outside for regular walks to meet new people. But the biggest reward has to be a pet's companionship and unconditional love.

458. GREAT EXPECTATIONS
Making lots of goals or over-committing yourself (when you might already be short on time) is a sure way of leaving you feeling inadequate when you don't achieve everything. Review the expectations you place on yourself and scrub some things off your To Do list.

459. FLOAT AWAY
Let go of stress by soaking in the bath or book a session in a flotation tank if you can! Weightlessness helps your body to let go of tension, which in turn influences your mind to relax. Studies show floating can create 'theta' brainwaves, which are associated with feelings of serenity which are normally achieved through deep meditation.

460. SIZZLING SEX
Don't let children, your job or domestic chores get in the way of your sex life. It has heaps of health benefits including helping depression, anxiety, insomnia and even prostate cancer in men. Squeeze in a quick sex session and release those endorphins to boost your mood.

461. SEEK SUN

Feeling gloomy? Getting out in the sunlight can cheer you up and help fight depression. If you work indoors or you're at home during the day, open curtains or blinds and turn on lights. Try to nip outside every now and then for 15 minutes or more. That's long enough to change chemicals in the brain to cheer you up and give you a blast of vitamin D for stronger bones.

462. BREATH OF FRESH AIR

Help treat anxiety and stress with deep breathing. Inhale slowly and deeply, filling your chest with air and count to four. (The count is to give you a nice and easy pace). Then breathe out slowly, again to the count of four. Repeat for five minutes when you feel under stress.

463. SWOT UP

Become an expert. There's great satisfaction to be gained from mastering a subject and it helps to build self-esteem. It can also lead to meeting others who share your interests. Pick a subject or hobby that interests you personally – be it 1950s fashion, cookery or Mozart.

464. SING SONG

Singing in the shower may be a cliché but it's a great way to start the day in a good mood. Belting out your favourite songs, either with music or without, releases tension and takes your mind off your troubles. Singing in the car can also be a good release for pent up frustration when you're stuck in a traffic jam.

465. SCRIBBLE AWAY

Keeping a diary or journal has a lot more benefits than people realize. As well as recording the happenings in your life, it helps you clarify your thoughts, release emotions and it can be a good problem-solving tool with worries that just won't go away.

466. NO GO

Learn to say no to people. If your friend asks you to baby-sit or your children try to rope you into helping them clear up, be assertive enough to say no. Taking on more than you can manage is a shortcut to stress, tiredness and low moods.

467. PICK A PAL

Mixing with friends and family or being part of a happy marriage is great for your mental and physical well-being. Studies show that spending time with a support network can boost your immune system and protect you from illness.

468. TICKTOCK

Going to bed and getting up at the same time every day keeps your sleep patterns regulated and that helps you sleep better. Adequate shuteye boosts your moods, energy levels and your looks.

469. SEEING RED

Colour therapy is based on the idea that specific colours are related to certain emotions. Everyday exposure to different colours can be achieved through the clothes you wear and the way you decorate your home. Colours have the following effects:

- red – stimulating and warming.
- yellow – increases intellect, creativity and mood.
- green – refreshing and calming.
- blue – soothing and cooling.
- white – cleansing and clarifying.
- black – oppressive and glamorous.

470. STRESS SOOTHER

Spinach is rich in magnesium, crucial for energy production and helping chronic fatigue problems. When your body's under stress your need for magnesium increases dramatically and studies show that the mineral supports our nervous system. Stick spinach in salads, sandwiches or serve it steamed with your main meal.

471. SORT IT OUT

You might think taking an hour to organize something, whether it's your desk or a closet, is a chore. But it can also be a stress reliever, especially if you're a perfectionist or somebody who gets bogged down in the small details of life. De-cluttering your surroundings will give you a sense of accomplishment and help you feel more in control.

472. STOP SNIFFLES

You've probably been told to take vitamin C when you've got a cold, but did you know zinc has become just as popular? Zinc is a mineral that plays a key role in regulating your immune system, helping wound healing and keeping skin healthy. You can find zinc in:

- seafood
- meat
- nuts
- dairy products
- wholegrains

473. POWER NAP

Are you sleep deprived and you don't know it? If you are you might be suffering from mood swings, low energy levels and increased cravings. A quick snooze of 20 – 30 minutes can work wonders to perk you up and help stress levels. But sleeping for longer interrupts your regular sleep cycle and will make you feel worse.

474. MONEY MATTERS

Studies show that depression and suicide rates are often linked to personal debt. Money worries affect most people to different extents. Pop into your local library or browse the Internet and you'll see there are plenty of charities and organisations set up to help people deal with debt. Get in touch and start sorting out your finances before it gets on top of you.

475. HEY GOOD LOOKING
The simple act of stopping and taking in a beautiful scene or object can improve your mood and reduce stress -whether you're gazing on a romantic sunset, glimpsing at a picture of a loved one or admiring a famous painting. They say the best things in life are free.

476. BEAT BOREDOM
A change is as good as a rest. If you're stuck in a rut give yourself a boost by changing your everyday routine - visit new places, do your shopping in a new town, change the route your walk your dog or take on a new challenge at work.

477. PIN-UP
Acupuncture is an ancient Chinese therapy with so much scientific research behind it that many GPs are recommending it instead of medication for a variety of health complaints. The treatment involves small pins being lightly pushed in to the top layer of your skin to stimulate your body's own healing process. It helps everything from stress and pain to skin conditions and bloating.

478. HAPPY PILLS
St John's Wort is a natural alternative to prescription anti-depressants. Studies show the yellow flower can help people with mild depression and anxiety. But taking it can increase sensitivity to sunlight, so slap on sun protection and see your GP first it if you're on other medications.

479. LOOK AFTER NUMBER ONE

Low self-esteem has been linked to depression and eating disorders. Learn to love yourself and focus on your good points instead of niggling doubts. Ask your GP to arrange for you to see a counsellor. They can help you go through underlying issues that might be contributing to the way you see yourself.

480. HEADS UP

Give yourself a head massage. Make small firm circles over your scalp, working from the front to the back of your head using your thumbs and fingertips. Concentrate particularly at the base of the head and around ears where tension builds up. Finish by lightly stroking all over your head.

481. WALK THIS WAY

Familiarize yourself with the Alexander technique. It teaches you how to sit, stand and move efficiently so you don't strain your body and you maximize your health. Benefits include better breathing, less painful joints and better moods. Find a local class to learn the basics.

482. HERB GARDEN

Plants were man's first medicine and many of today's medications are derived from them. You can buy herbal tea, tinctures, creams and capsules at health stores to treat a variety of conditions from stress to rheumatism. Most health stores have trained advisers who can answer your questions. But be careful because herbs can be potent. If you're pregnant or have any health problems then check with your GP first.

483. THE GREAT OUTDOORS

Stonehenge in England, Ayers Rock in Australia and Table Mountain in South Africa, there are numerous places of natural beauty all over the world that are said to have healing qualities. Whether or not they help your body isn't certain but they definitely help when you need some perspective on problems. But looking closer to home, simple things like listening to the wind blowing through the trees or water trickling down a stream can relax you.

484. GRIN AND BARE IT

Did you know that if you put on a false smile you'll actually begin to feel happier? Studies show that when people pretended to frown they started to feel angry, while the fake smilers felt happy. A big friendly grin is a great way of making a good first impression too.

485. PRESSING MATTER

Acupressure (basically acupuncture but without the needles, see tip 477) is based on the idea of using trigger points on your body to improve emotional and physical health. Slide your finger along the bone between the knuckle of your index finger and the joint where it comes down and connects to your thumb. Halfway along press into the fleshy mound and rub firmly. Repeat on the other hand. It's a handy exercise to tackle headaches and stress.

486. CHILD'S PLAY
Did you know children smile on average 400 times a day? While adults smile just 15 times? Be a child again and have a pillow fight, jump in puddles, take off your clothes and dance around the house (but maybe draw the curtains first!). It'll make you feel alive and youthful.

487. A TOUCH OF CLASS
Treating yourself to a bit of luxury can work wonders for bringing enjoyment into mundane chores. Buy a wonderful perfume, a lavish face cream or light some candles with your evening meal. Putting pleasure into little parts of your daily routine helps tackle boredom, depression and stress.

488. WHOLEMEAL FOR HEALTH
Next time you're at the supermarket have a quick scan over your trolley or basket and note how much white food you've got. Highly processed foods like white bread, pasta, sugar, rice and cakes are stripped of nutrients. Choose the wholemeal options instead and not only will you get more goodness but they'll keep you fuller for longer.

489. MAGIC MINERAL
Silica is hot news in skincare, the mineral found in barley, millet, oats, onions and wholewheat can increase the skin's elasticity and help store moisture and fight the signs of ageing.

490. ONE STEP BEYOND
Ginger promotes circulation and helps sweat out toxins. Treat yourself to an invigorating foot bath. Add 2tsps of ground ginger and 2tbsps of honey to a bowl of hot water. But before soaking your feet, inhale vapours under a towel if you have a cold to help to clear sinuses.

491. CHIN UP
Take a day off and do exactly what you want to do – and not what you think you should do. It'll fill you with renewed energy, boost your mood and give you time to do those little beauty jobs like a face pack, pedicure or get a new hair cut.

492. KITCHEN CURE
Tackle stress and anxiety by blending a drink that promotes calm and supports the nervous system. Mix up 2 romaine lettuce leaves, a handful of parsley, 4 carrots (with their tops removed) and 3 celery stalks.

493. SOLE MATE
Place both thumbs on the middle of the ball of your foot (the Solar Plexus) and lightly press and massage the area for a minute, then swap feet and do the same on the other food. It's a reflexology technique that's good for relaxation and tackling tension.

494. NO MORE NERVES
It's nice to get your glad rags on for a big event or party, but do you sometimes feel self-conscious and nervous about going? Get there early, it's easier to meet people when there are only a few guests and walking into a packed room of people already acquainted can make nerves worse.

495. LET OFF STEAM

Most sports centres, health clubs and gyms have saunas, for you to take full advantage of to relax and get rid of toxins. Just five minutes is enough to sweat out toxins and improve your skin. Avoid saunas if you're pregnant and seek medical advice before trying one out if you have existing medical conditions.

496. SMILES BETTER

Wholegrains and vegetables have long been an important part of a healthy diet. Experts say they contain B vitamins, which are vital for helping depression and other mental health problems. So stock up and help keep the blues at bay.

497. KEEP YOUR COOL

When you're about to explode or you're so stressed you could scream, think of somebody in your life who's cool-headed. It could be your mum or a friend from school. Then imagine how they would act in your shoes and use them as a positive role model.

498. PICTURE THIS

Looking at a cheerful screensaver on your computer will give you an instant lift. Download something brightly coloured from the Internet or scan in a picture that makes you smile. It makes your work day that bit more bearable.

499. UNFINISHED BUSINESS

Whether it's an urgent phone call you forgot to make or an unresolved argument, any unsolved problems are responsible for a third of insomnia cases according to studies. Before bed make a note of what's worrying you and what you want to do tomorrow. A list can make things seem more manageable and help you let go and drop off to sleep.

500. STRESS RELIEVER

Do something while you're relaxed and happy that you can repeat when you feel stressed to trigger a relaxed state. Pressing a certain part of your hand or pinging a wristband during a happy experience are popular techniques for making positive associations.

501. GO FOR IT

Remember it's never too late to do anything. Whether it's spending more time with family, learning a new skill, shaping up, going back to school, telling someone you love them or going on a holiday of a lifetime. Go and do something you've always dreamed of. Looking good starts on the inside, it's an attitiude to life.

Index